Cultural Practices
and Dermatoses

T0171902

Neelam A. Vashi
Editor

Cultural Practices
and Dermatoses

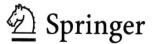 Springer

Editor
Neelam A. Vashi
Department of Dermatology
Boston University School of Medicine and Boston Medical Center
Boston, MA
USA

ISBN 978-3-030-68994-0   ISBN 978-3-030-68992-6   (eBook)
https://doi.org/10.1007/978-3-030-68992-6

This Springer imprint is published by the registered company Springer Nature Switzerland AG
The registered company address is: Gewerbestrasse 11, 6330 Cham, Switzerland

This book is dedicated to my greatest creations, Ethan and Ava, who will forever be my babies.

Preface

Cultural Practices and Dermatoses is a comprehensive text that examines specific dermatologic disease as it presents within a cultural context. As societies of the world become increasingly intertwined, both our local and far-reaching demographics diversify and cross-cultural exchange becomes commonplace. Physicians are rarely taught how cultural differences can affect disease presentation in patients. Without exposure to patients of varying backgrounds, it can be nearly impossible to learn about practices that may influence a patient's health. A well-known example of this in dermatology is mistaking cupping lesions as evidence of abuse. There are many more, less well-known examples of cultural practices causing dermatologic lesions, and it is becoming increasingly more likely that practicing dermatologists will encounter patients with these findings as migration, tourism, and public interest continue to rise. Patients are increasingly likely to try alternative therapies, particularly for chronic skin diseases. Dermatologists will need an understanding of the risks and benefits of these therapies in order to successfully counsel their patients.

Because of the breadth of knowledge that must be taught during medical school and residency, culture-specific disease findings are rarely included in curricula as compared with other topics. The practice of indigenous traditions is not limited to isolated territories. Dermatologists not studying or practicing in a highly multiethnic center may not be exposed to patients from many cultures. Although some cultural practices, such as acupuncture and threading, are widely used, there is limited medical literature describing their cutaneous effects and complications. This text aims to help dermatologists with the challenges involved in treating those from different backgrounds. I am forever grateful to my contributors for the hard work and dedication that were shared for this contribution to our dermatologic literature.

Boston, MA, USA   Neelam A. Vashi

Contents

Contributors

Casey C. Bunge, BA Department of Dermatology, Northwestern University Feinberg School of Medicine, Chicago, IL, USA

Nada Elbuluk, MD, MSc Department of Dermatology, Keck School of Medicine, University of Southern California, Los Angeles, CA, USA

Swati Garg, BA Department of Dermatology, Northwestern University Feinberg School of Medicine, Chicago, IL, USA

Roopal V. Kundu, MD Department of Dermatology, Northwestern University Feinberg School of Medicine, Chicago, IL, USA

Simone N. Montgomery, BA Department of Dermatology, Keck School of Medicine, University of Southern California, Los Angeles, CA, USA

Nicole Patzelt, MD Department of Dermatology, Boston Medical Center, Boston, MA, USA

Michelle Rodrigues, MBBS (Hons), FACD Royal Children's Hospital, Melbourne, VIC, Australia

Chroma Dermatology, Melbourne, VIC, Australia

Neda So, MBBS (Hons) BMedSc (Hons) MPHTM Royal Children's Hospital, Melbourne, VIC, Australia

Chroma Dermatology, Melbourne, VIC, Australia

Nicole Trepanowski, BS Boston University School of Medicine, Boston, MA, USA

Neelam A. Vashi, MD Boston University School of Medicine, Boston, MA, USA

Department of Dermatology, Boston Medical Center, Boston, MA, USA

Department of Dermatology, Boston University Center for Ethnic Skin, Boston, MA, USA

Boston University Cosmetic and Laser Center, Boston, MA, USA

Department of Veteran Affairs, Boston Health Care System, Boston, MA, USA

Chapter 1
Therapeutic Practices

Simone N. Montgomery and Nada Elbuluk

The 2012 National Health Interview Survey found that 33.2% of United States (US) adults and 11.6% of US children have used complementary alternative medicine (CAM) [1]. Use of CAM has been shown to contribute to delayed presentation and even non-utilization of biomedical treatment [2]. In some populations including those that are disproportionately affected by health disparities, CAM is often their first treatment choice, rather than seeking care from an allopathic physician, due to a multitude of access challenges and cultural barriers [3]. Many patients fail to share their use of CAM) with their health care providers in fear of anticipated disapproval [3]. This can be of particular concern given the danger of potential interactions with prescribed medications.

Familiarization of CAM practices is beneficial for all physicians including dermatologists. A review of numerous studies assessing CAM use by dermatology patients found a lifetime use between 35% and 69% [4]. Considering this, inquiry about CAM use to treat dermatological conditions should be incorporated into clinical history taking. Dermatologists must also be aware of the dermatological

S. N. Montgomery (✉) · N. Elbuluk
Department of Dermatology, Keck School of Medicine,
University of Southern California, Los Angeles, CA, USA

© The Author(s) 2021
N. A. Vashi (ed.), *Cultural Practices and Dermatoses*,
https://doi.org/10.1007/978-3-030-68992-6_1

adverse effects associated with CAM practices, which can include allergic and irritant contact dermatoses, bruising, and infections [5]. Additionally, while there is a growing breadth of peer-reviewed literature investigating CAM treatment options for dermatological conditions, there is a significant need for further investigation into the efficacy and adverse effects of CAM when used to (co)-treat dermatological conditions.

Increased use of CAM is seen across the US population, including in certain racial and ethnic groups, many of which are growing in number in the US. The greatest number of CAM therapies are derived from Asian countries. According to the 2010 Census, the Asian population is the most rapidly growing racial group in the US, and this trend is predicted to continue with the 2020 Census [6]. The number of people who identify as Asian is expected to reach 9.3%, or nearly 40 million, by the year 2050 [7]. "Asians" in the US are a highly diverse group stemming from the Far East, Southeast Asia, and the Indian subcontinent, with significant cultural diversity [8]. Many Asians share a deep connection with a variety of traditional CAM practices, many of which over time have been adopted by persons of all races worldwide. Considering the increased adoption of Asian CAM, this chapter will focus mainly on the more common traditional Chinese and other East Asian CAM practices and their dermatologic uses, efficacy, and adverse effects. These include traditional Chinese medicine, acupuncture, moxibustion, cupping, skin scraping techniques, Ayurvedic medicine, aromatherapy, gridding, salting, and toothpaste-associated treatments (Table 1.1).

Traditional Chinese Medicine

Originating in China over 3000 years ago, traditional Chinese medicine (TCM) employs a holistic approach to the body and mind with a focus on regulating the flow of Qi – the life force that flows throughout our body [9]. Qi flows through interconnected channels called meridians, and obstruction of

TABLE I.I Therapeutic practices, dermatological indications, and cutaneous adverse effects

Therapeutic practice	Common dermatological indications	Cutaneous adverse effects
Chinese herbal medicine[a]	Acne, alopecia areata, atopic dermatitis/eczema, bacterial/fungal infections, burns, chronic venous insufficiency, contact dermatitis, fungal infections Herpes simplex, Herpes zoster, hyperhidrosis, pruritus, psoriasis, scabies, seborrheic dermatitis, skin cancer, reactions, verrucae, vitiligo, wound healing [9, 12]	Acute generalized exanthematous pustulosis, allergic and irritant contact dermatitis, drug hypersensitivity syndrome, drug reaction with eosinophilia and systemic symptoms, erythema ab igne, pruritus, photosensitivity, Stevens-Johnson syndrome, toxic epidermal necrolysis [5, 12, 23, 24]
Needle acupuncture[a]	Acne, acute and chronic urticaria, alopecia areata, atopic dermatitis, herpes zoster, hyperhidrosis, impetigo, lichen planus, melasma, post-herpetic neuralgia, pruritus, rosacea, verrucae, vitiligo [5, 10]	Bleeding, bruising, foreign body granuloma, hematomas, Herpes simplex virus infection, keloids, koebnerization, local pain, prurigo nodularis, pyoderma gangrenosum, skin infection [12, 26]

(continued)

TABLE I.I (continued)

Therapeutic practice	Common dermatological indications	Cutaneous adverse effects
Moxibustion[a]	Alopecia areata, atopic dermatitis/eczema, post-herpetic neuralgia, psoriasis, scleroderma, tinea pedis, verrucae [30, 38–42].	First- and second-degree burns with subsequent scarring, targetoid patches [9, 43]
Cupping[a]	Acne, acute and chronic urticaria, atopic dermatitis/eczema, erysipelas, Herpes zoster, psoriasis, vitiligo [9, 12]	Bacterial infections, bullae, burns, circular petechiae, circular ecchymoses, circular purpura, erythema ab igne, hyperpigmentation, koebnerization, ulcers [12, 44, 45, 50, 52, 53]
Ayurveda	Acne vulgaris, molloscum contagiosum, psoriasis, vitiligo [10, 12]	Allergic and irritant contact dermatitis, burns, depigmentation [12]
Aromatherapy	Acne, alopecia areata, burns, contact dermatitis, eczema, Herpes infections, pruritus, psoriasis, radiation dermatitis, scarring, verrucae, wound healing, infections, xerosis [9, 67].	Allergic and irritant contact dermatitis, cheilitis, chemical leukoderma, perioral dermatitis, phototoxicity [12, 56]

TABLE 1.1 (continued)

Therapeutic practice	Common dermatological indications	Cutaneous adverse effects
Toothpaste	Burns, wounds [80]	Bacterial infection, oral cheilitis, slow wound healing, toothpaste-induced contact dermatitis (index finger) [75]
Skin scraping (*e.g.* coining, spooning)	None	Contact dermatitis, ecchymoses, edema, erythema ab igne, lichen planus pigmentosus, mild to severe burns, petechiae, purpura, ulcers [12, 43, 55, 57]
Gridding	None	Chemical burns, hyperpigmentation, maceration of skin [76, 77]
Salting	None	Epidermolysis, xerosis [79]

aConsidered a form of Traditional Chinese Medicine

these meridians is what is believed to cause pathology [5, 10]. A variety of TCM practices are used to decongest these channels and restore free flow of Qi [5]. TCM includes five traditional medical therapies: Chinese herbal medicine (CHM), acupuncture and moxibustion, therapeutic massage, meditative exercise practices, and dietary therapy [10–12]. Though TCM has been used for thousands of years throughout China and other East Asian countries, in recent decades its popularity has spread, and it is now widely practiced throughout the world [5, 11].

A survey of US adults between 1991 and 1997 found that 8.6% of respondents had used TCM for the management of dermatologic conditions, and considering the growing popularity of CAM, it is likely this number has since increased [13]. This increase in popularity of TCM is in large part owed to the growing interest in natural or homeopathic remedies as alternative or conjunctive treatment options to biomedical treatments. However, there is a significant lack of clinical trials and other studies investigating both the efficacy and potential adverse effects of these treatments. The growing presence of CAM and TCM practices is so significant that the National Institutes of Health have formed its own CAM institute to promote research in the field.

Chinese Herbal Medicine

Of particular importance in TCM is Chinese herbal medicine (CHM), or the use of unique combinations of medicinal herbs tailored for each individual patient [14]. The herbal remedies are used in pill, powder, teas, concentrate, topical ointment, and injection forms [12]. A significant amount of the available research on the use of CHM for the treatment of dermatologic disease involves use in atopic dermatitis and psoriasis.

TCM has a long history of use in the treatment of atopic dermatitis. First line TCM therapy for atopic dermatitis (AD) includes CHM preparations; acupuncture and moxibustion are also frequently used in conjunction for the treatment of AD [15]. There is limited evidence of improvement of erythema, affected surface area, and quality of life with oral herbal preparations [16–18]. In conjunction with Dr. Luo a Chinese physician and herbalist, Sheehan et al. conducted the first placebo-controlled, double-blind clinical trial investigating the use of CHM, for the treatment of AD [16]. An oral herbal treatment was prepared using multiple ingredients, including *Ledebouriella seseloides, Potentilla chinensis, Anebia clematidis, Rehmannia glutinosa, Paeonia lactiflora, Lophatherum gracile, Dictamnus ddsaycarpus, Tribulus terrestris, Glycyrrhiza uralensis,* and *Schizonepeta tenufolia,* and compared against a placebo mixture of inert agents with no known benefit in the treatment of AD [16]. Patients in the treatment group had a significant decrease of 91.4% of erythema and an 85.7% decrease in affected surface area, as compared to 10.6% and 17.3% decrease in the placebo group, respectively [16]. Another trial, which employed an oral, twice-daily concoction using *Flos lonicerae, Herba menthe, Cortex moutan, Rhizoma atractylodis,* and *Cortex phellodendri,* found CHM to be efficacious in reducing need for topical corticosteroid use as well as improving quality of life in a cohort of 85 children with moderate-to-severe atopic dermatitis [18].

Researchers estimate that 2% of patients with psoriasis in the US have been treated using CAM [19]. In Chinese medicine, psoriasis is believed to be a result of excess "evil heat" in the blood that stagnates in muscles and skin, eventually forming eruptions of dryness, pruritus, and scale [20]. Treatment of psoriasis is aimed at dissipating heat and cooling the blood [20]. Herbs used in the treatment of psoriasis are chosen for their anti-inflammatory and immunosuppressive effects, including *indigo naturalis, Tripterygium wilfordii, Tripterygium hypoglaucum,* and *Camptotheca acuminata* [9]. In one randomized, investigator-blinded, placebo-controlled clinical trial of 100 patients, a topical herbal treatment was proven to be significantly more effective at improving both investigator and subject assessment of psoriatic lesions, as compared to placebo, with no severe adverse effects [20]. *Indigo naturalis* has also been investigated for its effectiveness as an oral herbal monotherapy for the treatment of psoriasis. Investigators showed indirubin, the active ingredient in *Indigo naturalis,* to be more efficacious than ethyliminum [14]. A molecularly-modified derivative of indirubin is now widely sold throughout East Asia as a treatment for psoriasis. Treatments using furocoumarin-containing herbs, including *Radix angelicae dahuricae* and *Radix angelicae pubescentis,* are combined with UVA-phototherapy for a psoralen-like treatment effect for psoriasis [5, 9]. A multi-center study examining the use of the combination of *Radix angelicae dahuricae* with UVA phototherapy on over 200 patients showed a comparable treatment benefit to PUVA-phototherapy, with a mild adverse effect profile [21]. Although these results are encouraging, it is important to note that changes to participants' eye lenses have been reported with long-term use of *R. angelicae pubescentis* and UVA combination therapy [14].

Common side effects reported in CHM therapies include gastrointestinal side effects, transient elevations in liver function tests, and transient decreases in peripheral white blood cell counts [14, 22]. More severe adverse effects have rarely been documented, but include acute liver failure, dilated cardiomyopathy, and acute respiratory distress syndrome [12, 22]. Severe dermatological adverse reactions, including Stevens-Johnson syndrome/toxic epidermal necrolysis, drug hypersensitivity syndrome, acute generalized and exanthematous pustulosis, have also rarely been documented [5, 12, 23, 24].

While some clinical trials have shown efficacy in the management of certain dermatologic diseases, conducting randomized clinical trials is challenging given the individualized basis of CHM [12]. Because of this, there is little data comparing CHM against the more frequently used, first-line biomedical treatment options. Thus, there are significant concerns regarding the paucity of literature to investigate and characterize potential adverse effects and the true efficacy of these treatment options. These concerns are further complicated by the lack of standardized dose regulations for the use of medicinal herbs as medical treatments [25]. For example, in the US, medicinal herbs are classified as dietary supplements by the US Food and Drug Administration (FDA), and are thus not subject to the scrutiny of clinical trials [25]. Rates of contamination of products with medicines, like corticosteroids, acetaminophen, and others, have been estimated to be 4.5–23.7% [12]. Furthermore, many have been found to contain toxins, pesticides, and heavy metals [12]. Despite this, both oral and topical herbal treatments have become increasingly popular in the US as an alternative to biomedical treatment for the management of many dermatologic conditions. Further research is needed to ensure patients are able to use these alternative medicine techniques safely and effectively.

Needle Acupuncture

Needle acupuncture, or *Zhen Jiu*, is a popular TCM technique with an estimated use of 1.4% in US adults [12]. It is an ancient practice that is believed to have originated in China between 500,000 and 300,000 BC [12]. Sterile, fine needles are passed through the skin, subcutaneous tissue, and muscles to manipulate Qi and stimulate healing by relieving obstructions of the meridian channels that allow Qi to flow throughout our bodies [5]. There are over 2000 specific placement points on the skin, each of which is linked to a specific organ system [5]. Two styles are predominantly used; the Chinese style that includes manual stimulation of the needles and the Japanese style which does not [12].

Acupuncture has been used to treat numerous dermatologic conditions, including acne, alopecia areata, atopic dermatitis, herpes zoster, hyperhidrosis, impetigo, lichen planus, melasma, post-herpetic neuralgia, pruritus, psoriasis, rosacea, acute and chronic urticaria, verrucae, and vitiligo [5, 10]. Though there are numerous hypothesized mechanisms of action that have been suggested to explain the benefits of acupuncture for dermatologic disease, the exact mechanism of action has not been completely elucidated. Current hypotheses include stimulation of the hypothalamic pituitary-adrenal axis and/or other sensorineural pathways, including the autonomic nervous system, which subsequently stimulates the release of neurotransmitters and cytokines [9, 26, 27]. These pathways in turn lead to anti-inflammatory, anti-histamine, and immunomodulatory effects in the skin [9, 27].

There is significant evidence supporting the safety and efficacy of acupuncture in treating urticaria. Placebo studies have shown between 30% and 50% resolution of chronic urticarial lesions and up to 90% resolution in acute urticaria [27]. Furthermore, acupuncture has consistently been significantly more efficacious and resulted in a lower recurrence rate as compared to anti-histamines, which are considered one of the treatment mainstays for acute and chronic urticaria in the US [28, 29]. Acupuncture for the treatment of psoriasis is used throughout East Asia and is becoming more widely used throughout the world [30]. There are mixed results in investigations of acupuncture for the treatment of psoriasis. While some studies have found acupuncture to be a safe, beneficial treatment option for the management of psoriasis, a randomized clinical trial found acupuncture to be equivocal to sham acupuncture [31, 32]. However, many of the clinical studies investigating the use of acupuncture for the treatment of psoriasis are limited by sample size and adequate blinding, highlighting a need for future research to more rigorously investigate its benefits for patients with this condition [31, 32]. Atopic dermatitis and the benefits of acupuncture have also been reported. A randomized preliminary trial found that compared to sham-acupuncture placebo, acupuncture significantly improved Eczema Area and Severity Index score, patient pruritus, and quality of life in patients with mild-to-moderate atopic dermatitis [33]. Despite these encouraging findings in urticaria, psoriasis, and atopic dermatitis, more clinical studies and randomized clinical trials are needed to conclusively establish acupuncture as an efficacious treatment option for the management of dermatologic disease.

While fewer studies have investigated the treatments of dermatologic diseases directly, many studies have assessed the palliative effects of acupuncture on the symptoms of these disorders, including pain and pruritus [9]. For instance, there are identified placement points (such as *Qu Chi*, a specific placement point that is stimulated for the management of pruritus) that result in reduction of these symptoms, which can significantly improve one's quality of life, despite the persistence of the physical signs of the dermatological disorder. Multiple randomized clinical trials have shown significant reduction in both atopic dermatitis-induced and experimentally-induced histamine-related itch through the stimulation of Qu Chi and other points [26, 34, 35].

Acupuncture is considered safe with low risk of adverse effects when performed by trained practitioners. Common adverse effects occur at the needle-placement sites, including local pain, bleeding, bruising, and hematomas [26]. Other less common adverse effects include pneumothorax, spinal cord injury, anaphylactic shock, and organ puncture, though these are considered rare [12, 26]. Also considered rare are the adverse dermatologic manifestations, which include skin infections and the development of granulomas at needle-placement sites [26].

Moxibustion

Moxibustion is a TCM practice that has been used in East Asian countries for more than 4000 years [5, 36]. Many consider moxibustion a form of non-needle acupuncture [37]. The therapy involves burning pieces of the herb *moxa* on specific acupuncture points to decongest meridians and restore the flow of Qi [5, 36]. *Moxa* is an herb derived from the plant *Artemisia vulgaris,* more commonly known as mugwort. There are two moxibustion techniques, direct and indirect, both of which produce the desired effect. In the direct form, *moxa* cones are burned directly on the skin and removed only after pain is felt from the burning herb; in the indirect form, the *moxa* is placed on the tip of an inserted acupuncture needle or other insulating material and never comes into direct contact with the skin [5, 12]. Moxibustion is often used in combination with acupuncture for increased efficacy [36]. In the management of dermatologic conditions, the hypothesized mechanism of action is that the heat transferred from moxibustion improves local microcirculation and relaxes the epidermis in the treated areas [30].

Moxibustion has been studied for the treatment of alopecia areata, atopic dermatitis, post-herpetic neuralgia, psoriasis, scleroderma, tinea pedis, and verrucae [30, 38–42]. However, research is limited, and much of the literature consists of case reports and case series with a paucity of randomized clinical trials. Though moxibustion has shown to be a promising, safe, and beneficial treatment option in these dermatologic conditions, there is insufficient rigorously researched evidence that conclusively evaluates its efficacy.

Adverse effects of moxibustion are for the most part mild. Some patients report headaches, abdominal pain, or fatigue from smoke inhalation [12]. First- and second-degree burns with subsequent scarring are the most common long-term adverse effects, but occur infrequently [5, 9]. Transient targetoid patches, which may resemble cigarette burns, can also be present after treatments [12, 43]. The targetoid lesions and burns of moxibustion treatments can resemble physical abuse. For this reason, it is important that dermatologists are aware of these adverse effects and inquire about traditional health practices when patients present with these cutaneous manifestations.

Cupping

Cupping is an ancient therapy that aims to release excess "fire wind" (pain) [5] (Table 1.2). While traditionally cupping has been linked to TCM, there is evidence of its use in both ancient Greek and Egyptian civilizations [12, 44]. In more recent years, cupping has gained significant popularity as a form of CAM, especially after many prominent athletes promoted the benefits of its use during the 2016 Olympics [44].

The two most common types of cupping are the dry and wet technique. In dry cupping, a candle or burning alcohol is used to heat the air and consume the oxygen within the glass cup. The cup is then placed on the skin, creating a vacuum on the skin that draws blood and toxins to the surface of the skin [5, 12, 45]. More modern techniques use a handheld pump or

TABLE 1.2 Cupping techniques, considerations, and adverse effects

Cupping technique	Description	Adverse effects	Special considerations
Dry	A thick glass coated with burning alcohol is used to create a vacuum on skin.	Petechiae, ecchymoses, purpura	
Wet	Similar to dry cupping, with added technique of bloodletting.	Blood loss	Blood loss stimulates erythrocyte and leukocyte production in the bone marrow
	CPC method: Cupping is performed first, followed by puncturing the skin, and finished with second round of cupping. More commonly used in Middle East		Improves circulation by reducing blood viscosity
	PC method: Skin is first punctured followed by cupping. More commonly used in China, Korea, and Germany.		
Moving	Form of dry cupping that incorporates strokes of movement	Increased pain	Considered one of most effective

(continued)

TABLE 1.2 (continued)

Cupping technique	Description	Adverse effects	Special considerations
Needle	Form of wet cupping that incorporates oil and acupuncture	Increased risk of infection	Considered most effective for treatment of knee and elbow joints
Herbal	Form of dry cupping in which cups are first boiled with herbal remedies	Increased risk of burns	Herbal remedy is tailored to patient (similar to CHM); Performed with bamboo cups
Water	Cup is filled with water prior to placement on skin	Reduced bruising	Frequently used in children; Considered most effective for asthma and coughing
Pulsatile	Form of dry or wet cupping in which a pump is used to create a pulsatile vacuum		Considered most effective for large joints
Flash	Form of dry cupping in which cups are applied and then quickly removed		Often used when other forms are not tolerated

References [44–46]

vacuum to create the same effect [9]. When the cups are removed, circular petechiae, ecchymoses, and purpura remain, signifying the removal of toxins and inflammation from the body [5, 12]. Wet cupping, or *hijama*, is similar to dry cupping but adds a bloodletting component, in which the skin is punctured to physically draw up and release blood when the cup is placed on the skin [44]. The additional release of blood is believed to reduce viscosity and improve blood flow, as well as stimulate bone marrow production of erythrocytes and leukocytes [44]. Other types include moving cupping, needle cupping, herbal cupping, water cupping, pulsatile cupping, and flash cupping [44–46].

Dermatological indications for cupping include acne, atopic dermatitis, erysipelas, herpes zoster, psoriasis, acute and chronic urticaria, and vitiligo. One large systematic review of randomized clinical trials found that wet cupping was significantly more efficacious in curing, improving symptoms, and reducing complications of herpes zoster than traditional medical management [47]. A clinical trial of 38 patients with moderate acne vulgaris found wet cupping therapy to be a beneficial treatment [48]. Cupping has also been used successfully as an epithelial graft technique for the treatment of recalcitrant vitiligo. In a study of 20 patients, this technique resulted in repigmentation in over 80% of patients [49]. While the current literature reflects significant treatment benefits for these dermatological conditions, there are few randomized clinical trials and many of the remaining studies are limited by a lack of power due to small sample sizes [44, 45].

The most common adverse effects of cupping are cutaneous manifestations, including discrete circular, and occasionally linear, petechiae, ecchymoses, purpura, and burns [45, 50]. Similar to moxibustion, these findings are often mistaken for physical abuse [43]. Thus, it is important that dermatologists are aware of the dermatologic morphologies associated with cupping and inquire about patient TCM practices prior to considerations of physical abuse [9, 51]. Burns, bacterial infections, ulcer formation, hyperpigmentation, erythema ab igne, koebnerization and subsequent psoriatic plaque formation, and bullous pemphigoid eruptions are cutaneous adverse effects that have been less commonly reported [12, 44, 52, 53]. Additionally, anemia, panniculitis, and herpes viral infections are commonly seen in patients undergoing wet cupping therapy [50].

Skin Scraping: Spooning (*Guasha*) and Coining (*Cao gio*)

Skin scraping, also known as spooning or coining, is a CAM technique that originated in Vietnam and China and is used throughout East and Southeast Asia [12, 54]. *Gua sha*, or spooning, is a traditional Chinese form of linear dermabrasion using a Chinese soup spoon to release "excess wind" [55]. *Cao gio*, or coining, directly translates to "scrape wind." It is similar to spooning in both aim and technique, but employs a worn coin rather than a spoon and requires the treated area be lubricated with oils, ointments, or balms prior to scraping [55]. Though spoons and coins are traditionally used, skin scraping can be performed using any smooth-edged, ovoid object. Anecdotally, metal caps, animal bones/horns, jade, and ginger root have been used to perform the therapy [12]. Scraping is performed in a pine-tree formation until symmetric, linear striations are produced, which are believed to represent the release of the body's excess wind [54, 56]. The proposed mechanism of action is related to the dilation of capillaries, which is believed to result in release of impurities and excess heat and in the increased circulation of fresh blood [12, 54].

Skin scraping is believed by practitioners to be efficacious in the treatment of upper respiratory infections, musculoskeletal pain, headaches, seizures, febrile illness, and gastrointestinal disorders [12, 54]. While there are no reports of the use of skin scraping for the treatment of dermatologic disease, the potential dermatologic presentations that occur after therapy are relevant. The most common adverse effects of treatment are transient edema, petechiae, ecchymoses, and purpura that signify effective application of the therapy [55]. Similar to moxibustion and cupping, these cutaneous manifestations are frequently mistaken for physical abuse [5]. Mild burns, contact dermatitis, lichen planus pigmentosus, and systemic toxicity from the use of topicals, heated oils and ointments have also been reported as less common cutaneous adverse events [5, 12, 57]. It is important to note that there is one case report of a woman who sustained partial- and full-thickness burns on 22% of her body surface, requiring auto-grafting after the oils used during her coining therapy caught fire. Additionally, there is one report of cerebellar hematoma with subsequent herniation [12]. However, for most patients, the adverse effects of skin scraping are mostly transient and mild.

Ayurveda

Ayurveda, which translates directly to "the science of life," is an ancient system of healing that was first practiced over 5000 years ago in India and is considered India's equivalent to TCM [10, 12]. It is estimated that over 80% of the Indian population uses Ayurvedic medicine, and more recently Ayurvedic medicine has gained significant popularity in Western cultures [58]. A national survey reported that over 750,000 US adults have been treated by an Ayurvedic practitioner [58].

The basis of Ayurveda is balance of the three *doshas*, or forces – "*vaata*," "*pitta*," and "*kapha*" [12]. *Vaata* is believed to regulate the nervous system and movement, *pitta* is responsible for digestion and metabolism, and *kapha* controls strength and lubrication [10]. Illness is caused by any imbalance of the three *doshas*; thus, treatment is aimed at restoring each person's unique *dosha* equilibrium [10, 56]. Ayurvedic medicine incorporates four forms of therapy: herbal medications, oil massages, diet and lifestyle changes, and evacuative procedures (*e.g.* bloodletting) [10, 12].

Ayurveda has been used anecdotally to treat numerous dermatological diseases, including acne vulgaris, molluscum contagiosum, psoriasis, and vitiligo [10, 12]. However, the literature supporting the efficacy and safety of traditional Ayurvedic remedies remains limited. A randomized, double-blind clinical trial of 82 Indian patients with moderate acne vulgaris investigated the efficacy of four common oral Ayurvedic acne medications as compared to a placebo. Patients taking the Ayurvedic medication *Sunder Vati* were found to have a significant reduction in acneiform lesions as compared to placebo and the three other herbal formulations [59]. A case series of three patients with molluscum contagiosum reported accelerated resolution of symptoms following treatment with topical *Pratisaraniya Knara* and oral *Bilvadi Agada,* which are two Ayurvedic medicinal preparations [60]. Ayurvedic management of psoriasis has been more rigorously investigated. Studies have demonstrated the efficacy of curcumin (turmeric root), neem tree back (*Azadirachta indica*), and other Ayurvedic compound preparations [10, 61–64]. By measuring phosphorylase kinase activity, one study demonstrated that curcumin may even have greater efficacy in the treatment of psoriasis than calcipotriol [62].

There is a growing concern about the belief that the herbal remedies prescribed by Ayurvedic practitioners have no adverse effects because they are natural. However, common adverse cutaneous manifestations include burns, irritant dermatitis, and contact dermatitis [12]. Similar to the treatments used in CHM, the herbal treatments are classified as dietary supplements by the US FDA and are not as thoroughly regulated. Many of the commonly used herbs in Ayurvedic medicine have been shown to contain trace amounts of heavy metals, including arsenic, lead, mercury, and cadmium [65]. Furthermore, the levels of these metals can be significantly more elevated – some to even potentially toxic levels – when measured in Ayurvedic preparations [58, 66]. For example, one US study of Ayurvedic herbal remedies at a Bostonian market found that 20% of the sample contained heavy metal content that surpassed the upper limit of regulatory standards [66]. Given the paucity of literature on Ayurvedic medicine, it is important that further research be conducted to investigate both the efficacy and safety of this alternative herbal medicine.

Aromatherapy

Aromatherapy, also known as essential oil therapy, has its origin in several Asian cultures and encompasses the use of aromatic essential oils for therapeutic healing [67]. More recently, its use has gained significant popularity worldwide [68]. The aromatic herbal remedies used in traditional TCM and Ayurvedic therapies provide the foundation of this practice [67]. Oils are extracted by steam distillation or by cold pressing the leaves, stems, flowers, fruits, or roots of the plants, and then combined with other organic additives, including alcohols, aldehydes, aromatic aldehydes, ketones, esters, lactones, phenols, and terpenes [9].

There are many external and internal uses of essential oils in aromatherapy, though oral formulations are less commonly utilized [67]. While essential oils are most commonly used as oils for therapeutic massage or used in aerosolized form for inhalation, the list of alternative preparations includes baths, compresses, wound dressings, sprays, baths, or alternatively in aerosolized form as a spray or inhalant [9, 56, 67]. Aromatherapy is used to treat many medical conditions; the dermatological uses include acne, alopecia areata, burns, contact dermatitis, eczema, herpes infections, pruritus, psoriasis, radiation dermatitis, scarring, verrucae, wound healing, wound infections, and xerosis [9, 67].

In one randomized, double-blind, controlled trial of 86 patients with alopecia areata, daily aromatherapy massage using thyme, rosemary, lavender, and cedarwood oils mixed with a jojoba and grapeseed base was found to be a safe and efficacious treatment [69]. In this study, 44% of patients in the treatment group showed improvement based on blinded assessment of sequential photographs, as compared to 15% in the control group. The study did not report percent regrowth or use of a previously validated scale [69]. Tea tree oil is anecdotally used for its anti-septic and anti-fungal properties. Multiple large, randomized, double-blinded clinical trials have been performed investigating these properties. For the treatment of onychomycosis, topical 100% tree oil has been shown to have comparable results for clinical assessment and culture cure with 1% clomitrazole [70]. Another single-blind clinical trial found that in the treatment of acne, 5% tea tree oil gel was comparable in efficacy to 5% benzoyl peroxide lotion [9, 71]. A recent systematic review reported that essential oils could be considered as alternative treatments for acne, MRSA decolonization, and fungal infections, but also emphasized that there is significant need for additional studies to more rigorously investigate efficacy and safety [72].

Aromatherapy is generally considered safe and has a low risk profile. Common adverse effects are dermatological manifestations, including irritant and allergic contact dermatoses. The most common essential oils associated with patch-test confirmed allergic dermatitis are ylang-ylang, lemongrass, jasmine, sandalwood, and clove oils [56, 73]. While not common, phototoxicity has been reported after use of citrus-derived essential oils with high psoralen and furocoumarin content [9, 56, 74]. Lastly, similar to the concerns about CHM and Ayurvedic medicines, many essential oils are not all regulated by the FDA and some have been found to be contaminated with heavy metals [12].

Gridding

Gridding is a practice to treat respiratory illness in Russian and Eastern European folk medicine [75]. Practitioners use iodine to paint a criss-cross, or grid-like, pattern on the patient's back [12, 75]. This is believed to relieve cough and congestion by warming the chest [76]. While most patients report a mild burning sensation where the iodine is placed, the practice is otherwise considered to be safe and well-tolerated [75]. Two case reports have raised concern that topical use of concentrated iodine can lead to chemical burns and maceration of skin [76, 77]. Furthermore, prolonged iodine use in infants has been linked to hypothyroidism [76]. However, there is no literature linking these adverse effects to the practice of gridding. Gridding has not been studied for the treatment of dermatologic disease.

Salting

Salting is a custom performed in traditional Turkish culture believed to deter evil spirits that cause sickness and death [12, 75]. The practice is used in neonates and involves intermittently scrubbing the entire body with table salt for at least 1 hour, which is believed to improve the health of the neonate's skin and deter spirits [12, 75, 78]. Most commonly, infants subjected to this therapy have few adverse effects, though they may present with dry, dehydrated skin [75]. Rarely, cases of epidermolysis, severe hypernatremia and seizures, and death due to skin absorption of sodium have been reported [75, 78, 79]. Salting has not been studied for the treatment of dermatologic disease.

Toothpaste-Related Therapy

Toothpaste for Wound Treatments

Toothpaste is used as a cultural folk remedy for wounds and burns in Greece and Iran due to the soothing cooling effect of menthol and the anecdotal belief that it may improve healing and relieve pain [75]. However, the abrasive ingredients contained in toothpaste may paradoxically slow wound healing and increase the risk of infection [75]. There is currently no literature investigating the beneficial or adverse effects of toothpaste as a remedy for wounds.

Toothpaste-Induced Dermatitis

Toothpaste-induced dermatitis is a rare phenomenon seen mostly in India and other Southeast Asian countries that presents as simultaneous contact dermatitis on the index finger and oral cheilitis [12, 80]. This occurs in patients who routinely use their index finger rather than a toothbrush to scrub toothpaste on their teeth [12, 80]. In a case series of three patients with this combination of symptoms, a patch test using their personal toothpastes compared against petrolatum was positive in each case, supporting the diagnosis of allergic contact dermatitis. Change of toothpaste and a short course of topical steroid resulted in complete resolution of symptoms [81].

Diagnosis of toothpaste-induced dermatoses is rare for three reasons. First, the oral mucosa is robust and is relatively resistant to irritants and allergens [81]. The second is the lower potential for sensitization of the ingredients in toothpaste. Toothpaste ingredients that have been reported to cause contact cheilitis and allergic contact dermatitis include cinnamic aldehyde, fluorides, flavoring agents like peppermint, fragrance mixtures, balsam of Peru, sodium lauryl sulfate, triclosan, and propylene glycol [81]. The final reason is a general lack of simultaneous presentation of patients with both symptoms, which suggests that this condition may be underdiagnosed [81].

Conclusion

As the United States becomes more racially and ethnically diverse, the usage of alternative therapeutic medicine is growing in scope and practice. CAM continues to become more popular and is increasingly practiced amongst many outside of the populations where it originated. Thus, it is important that dermatologists are aware of the common alternative therapies discussed in this chapter in order to properly counsel patients and provide culturally-competent care. Dermatologists should be familiar with the cutaneous manifestations associated with moxibustion, cupping, skin scraping, gridding, and salting. History of TCM practices should be taken during the medical visit. Certain conditions may clinically appear similar to physical abuse and therefore awareness of these practices and their subsequent clinical presentation is significant. Additionally, further research is needed to investigate the safety and efficacy of many of these alternative treatments in order to accurately counsel patients on their risks and benefits. While many dermatologists may educate their patients based on allopathic guidelines, it is critical to respect and understand the cultural beliefs and customs of each patient. This will not only strengthen the patient-physician relationship but also ensure that patients feel comfortable discussing their practices openly.

References

1. Key findings. National Center for Complementary and Integrative Health; 2017.
2. Shim JM, Schneider J, Curlin FA. Patterns of user disclosure of complementary and alternative medicine (CAM) use. Med Care. 2014;52(8):704–8.
3. Arthur K, Belliard JC, Hardin SB, Knecht K, Chen CS, Montgomery S. Reasons to use and disclose use of complementary medicine use – an insight from cancer patients. Cancer Clin Oncol. 2013;2(2):81–92.
4. Ernst E. CAM in dermatology: telling fact from fiction. Int J Dermatol. 2003;42(12):979–80.
5. Mizuguchi RS, Kelly PT, Susan C. Asian cultural habits and practices. Dermatology for skin of color. New York: McGraw-Hill Medical; 2009.
6. Hoeffel EM, Rastogi S, Kim MO, Shahid H. The Asian population: 2010. Washington, DC: United States Census Bureau; 2012.
7. Colby SL, Ortman JM. Projections of the size and composition of the U.S. population: 2014–2060. Washington, DC: United States Census Bureau; 2015.
8. Race. United States Census Bureau; 2019.
9. Kasprowicz S, Lio P. Complementary and alternative medicine. In: Bolognia J, Schaffer JV, Cerroni L, editors. Dermatology. 4th ed. Philadelphia: Elsevier; 2018.
10. Bhuchar S, Katta R, Wolf J. Complementary and alternative medicine in dermatology: an overview of selected modali-

ties for the practicing dermatologist. Am J Clin Dermatol. 2012;13(5):311–7.

11. Yu F, Takahashi T, Moriya J, Kawaura K, Yamakawa J, Kusaka K, et al. Traditional Chinese medicine and Kampo: a review from the distant past for the future. J Int Med Res. 2006;34(3):231–9.

12. Vashi NA, Patzelt N, Wirya S, Maymone MBC, Zancanaro P, Kundu RV. Dermatoses caused by cultural practices: therapeutic cultural practices. J Am Acad Dermatol. 2018;79(1):1–16.

13. Eisenberg DM, Davis RB, Ettner SL, Appel S, Wilkey S, Van Rompay M, et al. Trends in alternative medicine use in the United States, 1990–1997: results of a follow-up national survey. JAMA. 1998;280(18):1569–75.

14. Koo J, Desai R. Traditional Chinese medicine in dermatology. Dermatol Ther. 2003;16(2):98–105.

15. Shi ZF, Song TB, Xie J, Yan YQ, Du YP. The traditional Chinese medicine and relevant treatment for the efficacy and safety of atopic dermatitis: a systematic review and meta-analysis of randomized controlled trials. Evid Based Complement Alternat Med. 2017;2017:6026434.

16. Sheehan MP, Atherton DJ. A controlled trial of traditional Chinese medicinal plants in widespread non-exudative atopic eczema. Br J Dermatol. 1992;126(2):179–84.

17. Zhang W, Leonard T, Bath-Hextall F, Chambers CA, Lee C, Humphreys R, et al. Chinese herbal medicine for atopic eczema. Cochrane Database Syst Rev. 2005;(2):Cd002291.

18. Hon KL, Leung TF, Ng PC, Lam MC, Kam WY, Wong KY, et al. Efficacy and tolerability of a Chinese herbal medicine concoction for treatment of atopic dermatitis: a randomized, double-blind, placebo-controlled study. Br J Dermatol. 2007;157(2):357–63.

19. Landis ET, Davis SA, Feldman SR, Taylor S. Complementary and alternative medicine use in dermatology in the United States. J Altern Complement Med. 2014;20(5):392–8.

20. Yan Y, Liu W, Andres P, Pernin C, Chantalat L, Briantais P, et al. Exploratory clinical trial to evaluate the efficacy of a topical traditional Chinese herbal medicine in psoriasis vulgaris. Evid Based Complement Alternat Med. 2015;2015:719641.

21. Zhang GW. Treatment of psoriasis by photochemotherapy: a comparison between the photosensitizing capsule of Angelica dahurica and 8-MOP. Zhonghua Yi Xue Za Zhi. 1983;63(1):16–9.

22. Sheehan MP, Atherton DJ. One-year follow up of children treated with Chinese medicinal herbs for atopic eczema. Br J Dermatol. 1994;130(4):488–93.

23. Mochitomi Y, Inoue A, Kawabata H, Ishida S, Kanzaki T. Stevens-Johnson syndrome caused by a health drink (Eberu) containing ophiopogonis tuber. J Dermatol. 1998;25(10):662–5.
24. Lim YL, Thirumoorthy T. Serious cutaneous adverse reactions to traditional Chinese medicines. Singap Med J. 2005;46(12):714–7.
25. Rousseaux CG, Schachter H. Regulatory issues concerning the safety, efficacy and quality of herbal remedies. Birth Defects Res B Dev Reprod Toxicol. 2003;68(6):505–10.
26. van den Berg-Wolf M, Burgoon T. Acupuncture and cutaneous medicine: is it effective? Med Acupunct. 2017;29(5):269–75.
27. Iraji F, Saghayi M, Siadat A. Acupuncture in the treatment of chronic urticaria: a double blind study. Int J Dermatol. 2005;3(2). https://ispub.com/IJD/3/2/4196.
28. Zhao JQ, Ma TM. A meta-analysis of acupuncture therapy for chronic urticaria. Zhen Ci Yan Jiu. 2020;45(1):66–73.
29. Shi Y, Zhou S, Zheng Q, Huang Y, Hao P, Xu M, et al. Systematic reviews of pharmacological and nonpharmacological treatments for patients with chronic urticaria: an umbrella systematic review. Medicine (Baltimore). 2019;98(20):e15711.
30. Xiang Y, Wu X, Lu C, Wang K. An overview of acupuncture for psoriasis vulgaris, 2009–2014. J Dermatolog Treat. 2017;28(3):221–8.
31. Coyle M, Deng J, Zhang AL, Yu J, Guo X, Xue CC, et al. Acupuncture therapies for psoriasis vulgaris: a systematic review of randomized controlled trials. Forsch Komplementmed. 2015;22(2):102–9.
32. Gamret AC, Price A, Fertig RM, Lev-Tov H, Nichols AJ. Complementary and alternative medicine therapies for psoriasis: a systematic review. JAMA Dermatol. 2018;154(11):1330–7.
33. Kang S, Kim YK, Yeom M, Lee H, Jang H, Park HJ, et al. Acupuncture improves symptoms in patients with mild-to-moderate atopic dermatitis: a randomized, sham-controlled preliminary trial. Complement Ther Med. 2018;41:90–8.
34. Belgrade MJ, Solomon LM, Lichter EA. Effect of acupuncture on experimentally induced itch. Acta Derm Venereol. 1984;64(2):129–33.
35. Pfab F, Huss-Marp J, Gatti A, Fuqin J, Athanasiadis GI, Irnich D, et al. Influence of acupuncture on type I hypersensitivity itch and the wheal and flare response in adults with atopic eczema – a blinded, randomized, placebo-controlled, crossover trial. Allergy. 2010;65(7):903–10.

36. Stein DJ. Massage acupuncture, moxibustion, and other forms of complementary and alternative medicine in inflammatory bowel disease. Gastroenterol Clin N Am. 2017;46(4):875–80.
37. Chen Z, Zhou D, Wang Y, Lan H, Duan X, Li B, et al. Fire needle acupuncture or moxibustion for chronic plaque psoriasis: study protocol for a randomized controlled trial. Trials. 2019;20(1):674.
38. Zhang YM, Liu CH, Wang YC, Teng HL, Meng XL, Han XJ. Medicated thread moxibustion for alopecia areata: a case report. Medicine (Baltimore). 2019;98(44):e17793.
39. Zhong J, Lin C, Fang G, Li JJ, Chen P. Observation on therapeutic effect of plum-blossom needle combined with medicated thread moxibustion of traditional zhuang nationality medicine on postherpetic neuralgia. Zhongguo Zhen Jiu. 2010;30(9):773–6.
40. Yan XN, Zhang JR, Zhang CQ, Tian Q, Chen L. Efficacy observation on acupuncture and moxibustion combined with hot compress of TCM herbs for scleroderma. Zhongguo Zhen Jiu. 2013;33(5):403–6.
41. Yun Y, Shin S, Kim KS, Ko SG, Choi I. Three cases of cutaneous warts treated with moxibustion. Explore (NY). 2016;12(4):277–81.
42. Tian YS, Chen L, Ren ZW, Wang XY, Liang TY, Wang LS. Observation on therapeutic effect of medicinal moxa stick moxibustion for treatment of tinea pedis. Zhongguo Zhen Jiu. 2009;29(7):537–40.
43. Chua S, Chen Q, Lee HY. Erythema ab igne and dermal scarring caused by cupping and moxibustion treatment. J Dtsch Dermatol Ges. 2015;13(4):337–8.
44. Soliman Y, Hamed N, Khachemoune A. Cupping in dermatology: a critical review and update. Acta Dermatovenerol Alp Pannonica Adriat. 2018;27(2):103–7.
45. Cao H, Li X, Liu J. An updated review of the efficacy of cupping therapy. PLoS One. 2012;7(2):e31793.
46. Tian J. Electroacupuncture combined with flash cupping for treatment of peripheral facial paralysis--a report of 224 cases. J Tradit Chin Med. 2007;27(1):14–5.
47. Cao H, Zhu C, Liu J. Wet cupping therapy for treatment of herpes zoster: a systematic review of randomized controlled trials. Altern Ther Health Med. 2010;16(6):48–54.
48. Xu J, Lin R, Wang J, Wu Y, Wang Y, Zhang Y, et al. Effect of acupuncture anesthesia on acne vulgaris of pricking-bloodletting cupping: a single-blind randomized clinical trail. J Tradit Chin Med. 2013;33(6):752–6.

49. Awad SS. Chinese cupping: a simple method to obtain epithe-lial grafts for the management of resistant localized vitiligo. Dermatol Surg. 2008;34(9):1186–92; discussion 92–3.

50. Kim T-H, Kim KH, Choi J-Y, Lee MS. Adverse events related to cupping therapy in studies conducted in Korea: a systematic review. Eur J Integr Med. 2014;6(4):434–40.

51. Qin Y, Beach RA. Visual dermatology: beyond bruising: cupping in a North American context. J Cutan Med Surg. 2019;23(3):331.

52. Azizpour A, Nasimi M, Shakoei S, Mohammadi F. Bullous pem-phigoid induced by Hijama therapy (cupping). Dermatol Pract Concept. 2018;8(3):163–5.

53. Vender R. Paradoxical, cupping-induced localized psoriasis: a koebner phenomenon. J Cutan Med Surg. 2015;19(3):320–2.

54. Marion T, Cao K, Roman J. Gua sha, or coining therapy. JAMA Dermatol. 2018;154(7):788.

55. Tanner BS, Catanese C, Lew EO, Rapkiewicz A. Pitfalls in the interpretation of traumatic socioethnic practices. J Forensic Sci. 2016;61(2):569–72.

56. Kundu RV, Patterson S. Dermatologic conditions in skin of color: part I. Special considerations for common skin disorders. Am Fam Physician. 2013;87(12):850–6.

57. Yang G, Tan C. Lichen planus pigmentosus-like reaction to Guasha. J Cutan Med Surg. 2016;20(6):586–8.

58. Khandpur S, Malhotra AK, Bhatia V, Gupta S, Sharma VK, Mishra R, et al. Chronic arsenic toxicity from Ayurvedic medi-cines. Int J Dermatol. 2008;47(6):618–21.

59. Paranjpe P, Kulkarni PH. Comparative efficacy of four Ayurvedic formulations in the treatment of acne vulgaris: a double-blind randomised placebo-controlled clinical evaluation. J Ethnopharmacol. 1995;49(3):127–32.

60. Kalasannavar SB, Sawalgimath MP. Molluscum conta-giosum: a novel Ayurvedic approach. Anc Sci Life. 2013;33. India2013.:49–51.

61. Mangal G, Sharma RS. Clinical efficacy of Shodhana Karma and Shamana Karma in Mandala Kushtha (Psoriasis). Ayu. 2012;33(2):224–9.

62. Heng MC, Song MK, Harker J, Heng MK. Drug-induced suppres-sion of phosphorylase kinase activity correlates with resolution of psoriasis as assessed by clinical, histological and immunohis-tochemical parameters. Br J Dermatol. 2000;143(5):937–49.

63. Pandey S, Jha A, Kaur V. Aqueous extract of neem leaves in treatment of Psoriasis vulgaris. Indian J Dermatol Venereol Leprol. 1994;60(2):63–7.

64. Mehta CS, Dave AR, Shukla VD. A clinical study of some Ayurvedic compound drugs in the assessment quality of life of patients with Eka Kushtha (psoriasis). Ayu. 2011;32(3):333–9.

65. Nema NK, Maity N, Sarkar BK, Mukherjee PK. Determination of trace and heavy metals in some commonly used medicinal herbs in Ayurveda. Toxicol Ind Health. 2014;30(10):964–8.

66. Saper RB, Kales SN, Paquin J, Burns MJ, Eisenberg DM, Davis RB, et al. Heavy metal content of ayurvedic herbal medicine products. JAMA. 2004;292(23):2868–73.

67. Stevensen CJ. Aromatherapy in dermatology. Clin Dermatol. 1998;16(6):689–94.

68. Gupta D, Thappa DM. Dermatoses due to Indian cultural practices. Indian J Dermatol. 2015;60(1):3–12.

69. Hay IC, Jamieson M, Ormerod AD. Randomized trial of aromatherapy. Successful treatment for alopecia areata. Arch Dermatol. 1998;134(11):1349–52.

70. Buck DS, Nidorf DM, Addino JG. Comparison of two topical preparations for the treatment of onychomycosis: Melaleuca alternifolia (tea tree) oil and clotrimazole. J Fam Pract. 1994;38(6):601–5.

71. Bassett IB, Pannowitz DL, Barnetson RS. A comparative study of tea-tree oil versus benzoylperoxide in the treatment of acne. Med J Aust. 1990;153(8):455–8.

72. Deyno S, Mtewa AG, Abebe A, Hymete A, Makonnen E, Bazira J, et al. Essential oils as topical anti-infective agents: a systematic review and meta-analysis. Complement Ther Med. 2019;47:102224.

73. Uter W, Schmidt E, Geier J, Lessmann H, Schnuch A, Frosch P. Contact allergy to essential oils: current patch test results (2000–2008) from the Information Network of Departments of Dermatology (IVDK). Contact Dermatitis. 2010;63(5):277–83.

74. Kaddu S, Kerl H, Wolf P. Accidental bullous phototoxic reactions to bergamot aromatherapy oil. J Am Acad Dermatol. 2001;45(3):458–61.

75. Ravanfar P, Dinulos JG. Cultural practices affecting the skin of children. Curr Opin Pediatr. 2010;22(4):423–31.

76. Pappano DA. Gridding: a form of folk medicine for respiratory illness. Pediatr Emerg Care. 2009;25(9):603–4.

77. Lowe DO, Knowles SR, Weber EA, Railton CJ, Shear NH. Povidone-iodine-induced burn: case report and review of the literature. Pharmacotherapy. 2006;26(11):1641–5.
78. Yercen N, Caglayan S, Yucel N, Yaprak I, Ogun A, Unver A. Fatal hypernatremia in an infant due to salting of the skin. Am J Dis Child. 1993;147(7):716–7.
79. Swerdlin A, Berkowitz C, Craft N. Cutaneous signs of child abuse. J Am Acad Dermatol. 2007;57(3):371–92.
80. Ghosh SK, Bandyopadhyay D. Dermatoses secondary to Indian cultural practices. Int J Dermatol. 2014;53(4):e288–9.
81. Ghosh SK, Bandyopadhyay D. Concurrent allergic contact dermatitis of the index fingers and lips from toothpaste: report of three cases. J Cutan Med Surg. 2011;15(6):356–7.

Chapter 2
Cosmetic Practices

Swati Garg and Roopal V. Kundu

With greater globalization and immigration, cultural competency and cultural humility is becoming increasingly important in clinical settings. Cosmetic practices are extremely diverse and are often influenced by cultural perceptions of beauty. Recognizing the various cosmetic practices and their associated dermatoses that exist among cultures is imperative to ensure proper quality of care. Understanding the cultural implications behind practice will allow for better treatment options and a stronger relationship between the physician and patient. This chapter will cover the cultural practices of henna, threading, bindi and kumkum, sari drawstrings, decorative nose piercings, scarification, skin lightening, and cultural tattooing and their associated dermatoses.

Henna

Henna is a dye from the plant *Lawsonia Inermis* traditionally used in South Asian, Middle Eastern and African populations for cultural and cosmetic practices including temporary tat-

S. Garg · R. V. Kundu (✉)
Department of Dermatology, Northwestern University Feinberg School of Medicine, Chicago, IL, USA
e-mail: roopal.kundu@nm.org

© The Author(s) 2021
N. A. Vashi (ed.), *Cultural Practices and Dermatoses*,
https://doi.org/10.1007/978-3-030-68992-6_2

31

tooing or hair dye for weddings, holidays, ceremonies, and rituals [1]. Henna use has recently become popular in Western countries as a temporary tattoo, especially in tourist areas [2]. Lawsone is a compound found in natural henna that produces a temporary red pigment; thus natural henna is also referred to as "red henna". Most modern hennas, or "black henna", use p-phenylenediamine (PPD) as an additive to shorten the drying time and produce a black pigment [2]. PPD is a common ingredient in hair dyes and is a known sensitizer [3]. Other commonly found ingredients include heavy metals such as nickel (<2.5–3.96 ppm), cobalt (2.96–3.54 ppm), and lead (2.29–65.98 ppm) [4, 5]. Ingredients added to improve color or texture include coffee, black tea, lemon juice, eucalyptus, clove, mustard oil, vinegar, indigo powder, fenugreek seeds, okra, and tamarind paste [3, 6, 7]. A rarer form of henna known as henna stone is commercially sold as a solid material that is crushed into powder to make a black henna paste for temporary tattooing or hair dyeing [8]. PPD concentrations in henna stone (84.89–90.90%) [9] have been found to be significantly higher than those in black henna (2.35–29.5%) [4, 10, 11].

The most frequent complication from henna application is allergic contact dermatitis (ACD). ACD incidence at the site of henna application is thought to be as high as 2.35% [12]. However, few allergic cases have been reported due to natural red henna [6, 13]. Most complications of henna use arise from PPD exposure in black henna [1]; positive PPD patch tests have been reported in many cases of henna-induced ACD. PPD has also been found to cause airborne contact dermatitis from henna stone [14]. Sequelae of these reactions include hyperpigmentation, keloids, leukoderma, and permanent post-inflammatory hypopigmentation [15–18]. It is important to note that PPD is not the only compound associated with henna-induced ACD. One case reported a patch test positive for resorcinol as a rare allergen of black henna-induced ACD [19]. In addition, reported instances of ACD had patch tests negative for PPD [20].

Other complications of henna use include contact urticaria, irritant contact dermatitis, erythema multiform-like reaction, temporary hypertrichosis, superficial epidermal necrosis, lichenoid reactions, pigmented contact dermatitis, and angioedema [3, 12, 15, 16, 21–24]. Henna use has also been associated with many systemic and life-threatening complications. Multiple cases of life-threatening hemolysis in children with glucose-6-phosphate dehydrogenase deficiency secondary to henna usage have been reported [25, 26]. It is believed the structural similarity of lawsone to the oxidant 1,4-naphthoquinone accounts for hemolysis in G6PD deficient patients [26]. Rare instances of acute kidney injury, angioedema, and acute compartment system have been associated with henna use [21, 27, 28]. One case reported severe upper airway obstruction following ingestion of PPD in henna stone solution, eventually requiring emergency tracheotomy [29]. Hairdressers and artists are at higher risk to henna complications due to occupational exposure. One study found that 3.2% of Indian beauticians had positive patch tests to henna mixture [30].

Patients experiencing complications from henna are advised to avoid henna products containing PPD [1]. Pure henna is a safer alternative and should be used instead of black henna.

Threading

Threading (*bande abru* in South Asia, *khite* in Arabic, *fatlah* in Egypt) is a form of temporary hair removal common in South Asian and Middle Eastern countries but is gaining popularity globally for its affordability, precision, tolerability, and efficiency [1, 31]. Hair removal utilizing threading is most common on the cheeks, forehead, or ears for men and on the eyebrows, cheeks, chin, and upper lip for women [32]. Hairs are enclosed in an open loop of thread that is secured by the operator. The operator closes the loop of thread with their hands in a rapid, tight motion to trap the hair in the loop of thread and pull the entire hair shaft out. Tension is maintained on the thread by having the operator tie the thread around their neck or holding it in one's mouth. High cotton thread tends to grip hair better and are preferred to synthetic thread. Mild pain is often reported with threading [33]. Facial threading has been found to reduce skin roughness, producing an effect similar to exfoliation [31].

Although threading is considered relatively safe, there are complications associated with this epilation technique. Common complaints include pruritus, erythema, edema, irritant dermatitis, and dyspigmentation at the site of hair removal [13, 32, 33]. Dermatoses associated with threading include bullous impetigo, folliculitis, pseudofolliculitis, verrucae, koebnerized vitiligo, and molluscum contagiosum [32, 34–39]. Sequelae of bullous impetigo include post-inflammatory hyperpigmentation [32]. Reported cases of verrucae have resulted from both direct infection after threading and koebnerization of human papillomavirus from an initial lesion elsewhere on the body [34, 35, 38]. Although rare, damage to the skin barrier during threading increases the risk of infection [38, 40]. Potential sources of contamination include the thread, the operator's hands or mouth, cotton balls, and powder applied during threading [38, 40]. Undesirable effects of threading are highly dependent on the skill of the operator and the extent of skin abrasion from the thread movement [35]. Aseptic technique should be practiced by the operator to decrease infectious sequelae; this includes cleaning the area to be treated, avoiding placing the thread in the operator's mouth, and using sterilized single-use thread [40, 41].

Bindi and Kumkum

Bindi and Kumkum are commonly worn by Hindu women as a decorative adornment to the forehead (Fig. 2.1). Traditionally, they were used as a symbol of marital status but have since been popularized as a decorative cosmetic. The terms Kumkum and bindi are often used interchangeably but are not synonymous. Kumkum is applied as a paste or powder in a reddish color, and traditionally prepared at home with turmeric powder [42]. Current preparations have been found to include coal tar dyes, toluidine red, erythrosine, lithol red calcium salt, lead oxide, fragrances, groundnut oil, tragacanth gum, parabens, canaga oil, sandalwood, thimerosal, propyl gallate, PPD, Sudan-1, Brilliant Lake Red R, and aminoazobenzene [42–49]. Bindi is usually applied as a self-stick adhesive (Fig. 2.2), though a paste form is also available [42]. Compounds found in bindi include gallate mix, thimerosal, nickel, polyvinylchloride, PPD, tert-butyl hydroquinone, aminoazobenzene, Disperse Blue 124, Disperse Blue 106 [44, 45, 50, 51].

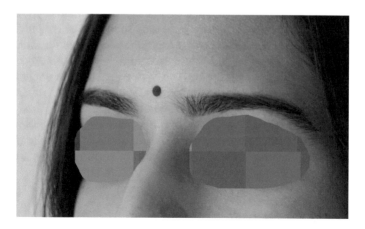

FIGURE 2.1 Adhesive Bindi worn on the forehead

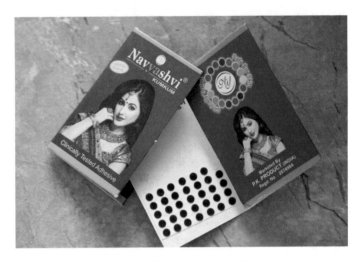

<small>FIGURE 2.2</small> Packets of self-stick adhesive Bindi

Contact leukoderma is a common complication reported from adhesive bindi use [52–55]. Para-tertiary-butylphenol (PTBP) has been found in bindi adhesive material but patch tests reveal PTBP is not the source of hypersensitivity [52, 53]. Bajaj reports all subjects in a study showed positive patch tests to the adhesive side of the bindi [56]. Depigmentation is likely attributed to individual susceptibility or prolonged bindi use [52, 53]. Other dermatoses reported include allergic contact dermatitis, pigmented contact dermatitis, contact vitiligo, lupus vulgaris, hyperpigmentation, and foreign body granuloma formation [51, 57–62]. Contact dermatitis often presents as erythema with papules and vesicles at the site of bindi application [61]. Individuals with adverse reactions are advised to discontinue use of bindi and Kumkum.

Sari Drawstrings

South Asian traditional clothing such as saris and salwaars contain drawstrings to secure the clothing around the waist. Saris are a single piece of fabric, typically 6 yards long,

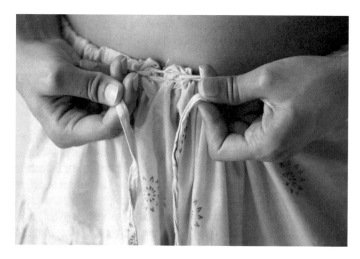

FIGURE 2.3 Traditional salwar with drawstring

draped around the body with an underlying petticoat containing the drawstring [1]. Salwaar is the lower trouser portion of the "salwar kameez" trouser and tunic combination [63]; salwaars are secured to the abdomen with a drawstring (Fig. 2.3).

Drawstring complications result from a combination of chronic friction, humidity, sweat, and abdominal folds [63]. Chronic frictional pressure from the drawstring can create a lichenified and hyperkeratotic band of hyperpigmentation [1, 63].The skin where the drawstring is tied is prone to koebnerization of pre-existing vitiligo and lichen planus (LP) [63]. Koebnerization of vitiligo and LP has been reported from friction of sari drawstring use [64, 65]. Given the relative humidity at the abdominal location, sweating and obesity at the drawstring line lead to an opportunity for secondary cutaneous infection by bacteria and fungi. Locally induced inflammation may also contribute to pruritus, irritant dermatitis, or allergic contact dermatitis [63]. In rare cases, similar to Marjolin's ulcer seen in chronic wounds or scars, a form of squamous cell carcinoma called "sari cancer" can occur from the chronic friction [63]. Patients are advised to tie the drawstring less tightly to reduce the amount of friction, especially those predisposed to vitiligo, LP, or other dermatological conditions [41].

Decorative Nose Piercings

Cosmetic nose piercing originated in the Middle East over 4000 years ago and has since gained worldwide prevalence [66]. Decorative nose piercings carry a cultural significance in many South Asian countries because they are often worn by the bride at marriage ceremonies [1]. The piercings generally consist of non-allergenic metals such as stainless steel, gold, niobium, and titanium but can contain allergens such as nickel [67].

Complications from nose piercings include allergic contact dermatitis, infection, keloid formation, scarring, bleeding, and collapse of the nasal wall [67, 68]. Post-piercing complications include infections most commonly due to *Staphylococcus aureus, Pseudomonas aeruginosa, Mycobacterium tuberculosis, Streptococcal pyogenes,* atypical mycobacteria, along with viral hepatitis [67–69]. Systemic infective endocarditis is a rare but reported sequela [68, 69]. Rare cases of pyogenic granuloma persistent telangiectatic erythema, and basal cell carcinoma as complications of nose piercing have been reported [69–71]. Nonsterile instruments, improper technique, non-hygienic standards, and inadequate post-piercing care pose a higher risk of developing complications [68].

Scarification

Scarification is the process of intentionally creating superficial scars on the skin using a knife, razor blade, stone, or glass [72]. This practice is commonly seen in African societies for therapeutic purposes and cultural expression such as community status, passage into adulthood, or spiritual or tribal identity [72, 73]. Therapeutic efficiency has not been proven with scarification [73]. Although prevalence of scarification is decreasing, it still remains popular in some traditional societies [74].

The most common complication associated with scarification is keloid formation, and often this is the desired effect [1]. Scarification has been associated with HIV, hepatitis B, hepatitis C, filarial elephantiasis, squamous cell carcinoma, and sarcoidosis [75–79]. Sterile technique should be practiced to decrease the risk of infectious sequelae [80].

Skin Lightening

Skin lightening practices are commonplace in Asia, Africa, the Caribbean, the Middle East, South America, Central America, Europe, and North America [81–86]. Prevalence of skin lightening is reported anywhere from 26% in Senegal to 75% in Nigeria [86]. Skin lightening practices are widely used by darker skinned patients for cosmetic enhancement often related to the cultural belief that a lighter skin tone is more attractive. There may also be cultural implications such as increasing prospects for marriage or representing a higher caste [86].

The composition of skin lightening creams is extremely variable within and between countries. Ingredients used in these creams are often prohibited or obtained illegally [81]. The standard skin lightening ingredient is hydroquinone however the compound is banned in many countries including the European Union and Japan [87]. Other compounds that have been found in topical skin lightening products include corticosteroids, glutathione, mequinol, retinoids, azelaic acid, arbutin, kojic acid, aleosin, licorice extract, ascorbic acid, N-acetyl glucosamine, sodium metabisulfite, kojic acid, 5,5′-dipropylbiphenyl-2,2′-diol, phenylethyl resorcinol, 3-o-ethyl ascorbic acid, lemon juice, potash, toothpaste, methyl gentisate, peroxides, and chlorates [1, 87–93]. Heavy metals are common additives in skin lighteners. Most concerning is the presence of mercury in these products [94]. One study found the prevalence of mercury above 1000 ppm in skin lighteners to be 6.0%, with some estimates reported as high as 16% [94]. Other metals found in these products include nickel, lead, chromium, cobalt, manganese, copper, aluminum, iron and zinc [84, 95], often in excess of recommended safety limits.

Up to 75% of individuals using skin lighteners have reported associated complications, with the degree of side effects experienced often correlating with the duration of product usage [96]. Because of the variability in the composition of skin lighteners, it can be difficult to deduce the specific effects of each component. Contact dermatitis from skin lightener usage has been attributed to numerous ingredients including but not limited to hydroquinone, sodium metabisulfite, kojic acid, 5,5'-dipropylbiphenyl-2,2'-diol, phenylethyl resorcinol, licorice extracts, and arbutin [88–91, 97–99]. More serious or systemic complications include leukoderma, toxic epidermal necrolysis-like chemical burns, tinea infection, corneal or scleral pathology, and squamous cell carcinoma [85, 100–103].

Specific complications are associated with the three most common classes of skin lightening ingredients: hydroquinone, corticosteroids, and mercury derivatives. Exogenous ochronosis is the most permanent complication of hydroquinone use in skin lighteners [104] Given their secondary bleaching effect, topical corticosteroids may be incorporated into skin lighteners and used unknowningly for prolonged periods of time. Extended use of corticosteroids for skin lightening can lead to skin atrophy, dermatitis, folliculitis, and rosacea [104]. Mercury is known to cause numerous neurologic, neonatal, and renal toxicities including paresthesia, respiratory distress, numbness, ataxia, and seizures. Concentrations of mercury in skin lightening products are often above recommended limits, making mercury complications more likely [1]. 45% of a sample of mercury-containing skin lighteners were found to contain over 10,000 ppm of mercury, well in excess of the FDA's limit of 65 ppm [94].

Cultural Tattooing

Ritual tattooing is a permanent pigment implantation into the skin for cultural purposes [1]. Many religions, particularly Hinduism and Buddhism, use tattooing as a way to manifest devotion, represent protection against evil, or symbolize identification with a group [74, 105]. One example is the practice of gingival tattooing in Ethiopian culture where a blue pigment is introduced to the gingiva through a needle [106].

Up to 5% of tattoo recipients develop cutaneous infection complications from *Staphylococcus Aureus* or *Streptococcus Pyogenes* such as impetigo, cellulitis, erysipelas, or abscesses [107]. Other cutaneous complications include hyperpigmentation, allergic contact dermatitis to pigment, keloid formation, contact urticaria, and koebnerization [79, 108]. Systemic complications often arise from disseminated infection of hepatitis B, hepatitis C, and HIV due to non-sterile technique [107]. The risk of these infections remains higher in cultural and ritual tattooing where sterile technique is not regularly observed. Serious complications reported include spinal abscess, retinal vasculitis, endocarditis, uveitis, and systemic zygomycosis [79, 107, 108].

Conclusion

As cultural cosmetic practices such as threading and henna become more prevalent in Western countries, it is increasingly important that dermatologists are aware of the skin manifestations of these practices. Numerous pathologic consequences are associated with these techniques and require proper diagnosis and treatment. Furthermore, an understanding of cultural competency is essential for an effective physician-patient relationship. Identifying the diagnosis and treatment addresses the patient's physical problems but does not tackle the patient's health beliefs and practices. Cultural competency is an important step towards comprehensive patient care that begins with understanding various cultural practices.

References

1. Vashi NA, Patzelt N, Wirya S, Maymone MBC, Kundu RV. Dermatoses caused by cultural practices: cosmetic cultural practices. J Am Acad Dermatol. 2018;79(1):19–30.
2. Le Coz CJ, Lefebvre C, Keller F, Grosshans E. Allergic contact dermatitis caused by skin painting (pseudotattooing) with black henna, a mixture of henna and p-phenylenediamine and its derivatives. Arch Dermatol. 2000;136(12):1515–7.
3. Kazandjieva J, Grozdev I, Tsankov N. Temporary henna tattoos. Clin Dermatol. 2007;25(4):383–7.
4. Kang IJ, Lee MH. Quantification of para-phenylenediamine and heavy metals in henna dye. Contact Dermatitis. 2006;55(1):26–9.
5. Jallad KN, Espada-Jallad C. Lead exposure from the use of Lawsonia inermis (henna) in temporary paint-on-tattooing and hair dying. Sci Total Environ. 2008;397(1–3):244–50.
6. Polat M, Dikilitas M, Oztas P, Alli N. Allergic contact dermatitis to pure henna. Dermatol Online J. 2009;15(1):15.
7. Swan BC, Tam MM, Higgins CL, Nixon RL. Allergic contact dermatitis to substitute hair dyes in a patient allergic to para-phenylenediamine: pure henna, black tea and indigo powder. Australas J Dermatol. 2016;57(3):219–21.
8. Ozkaya E, Yazganoglu KD. Henna stone: a lesser-known solid material from which to obtain black henna paste. Contact Dermatitis. 2013;69(6):386.
9. Ozkaya E, Yazganoglu KD, Arda A, Topkarci Z, Ercag E. The "henna stone" myth. Indian J Dermatol Venereol Leprol. 2013;79(2):254–6.
10. Almeida PJ, Borrego L, Pulido-Melian E, Gonzalez-Diaz O. Quantification of p-phenylenediamine and 2-hydroxy-1,4-naphthoquinone in henna tattoos. Contact Dermatitis. 2012;66(1):33–7.
11. Al-Suwaidi A, Ahmed H. Determination of para-phenylenediamine (PPD) in henna in the United Arab Emirates. Int J Environ Res Public Health. 2010;7(4):1681–93.

12. Berih A, Berhanu A. Allergic dermatitis – black henna (para-phenylenediamine) use among the East African patient population in a general practice setting. Aust Fam Physician. 2014;43(6):383–5.

13. Gupta D, Thappa DM. Dermatoses due to Indian cultural practices. Indian J Dermatol. 2015;60(1):3–12.

14. Ozkaya E, Topkarci Z. Airborne allergic contact dermatitis caused by a henna stone. Contact Dermatitis. 2016;75(3):191–2.

15. Valsecchi R, Leghissa P, Di Landro A, Bartolozzi F, Riva M, Bancone C. Persistent leukoderma after henna tattoo. Contact Dermatitis. 2007;56(2):108–9.

16. Gunasti S, Aksungur VL. Severe inflammatory and keloidal, allergic reaction due to para-phenylenediamine in temporary tattoos. Indian J Dermatol Venereol Leprol. 2010;76(2):165–7.

17. Bukhari IA. Cutaneous hyperpigmentation following nonpermanent henna tattoo. Saudi Med J. 2005;26(1):142–4.

18. Wohrl S, Hemmer W, Focke M, Gotz M, Jarisch R. Hypopigmentation after non-permanent henna tattoo. J Eur Acad Dermatol Venereol. 2001;15(5):470–2.

19. Ormerod E, Hughes TM, Stone N. Allergic contact dermatitis caused by resorcinol following a temporary black henna tattoo. Contact Dermatitis. 2017;77(3):187–8.

20. Sivam A, Tankersley M. Allergic contact dermatitis to henna tattoo with negative patch to p-phenylenediamine (PPD). J Allergy Clin Immunol Pract. 2019;7(1):288–9.

21. Ngwanya RM, Spengane Z, Khumalo N. Angioedema, an unusual reaction to hair dye. Pan Afr Med J. 2018;30:103.

22. Woo YR, Kim JS, Lim JH, et al. Acquired diffuse slate-grey facial dyspigmentation due to henna: an unrecognized cause of pigment contact dermatitis in Korean patients. Eur J Dermatol. 2018;28(5):644–8.

23. Davari P, Maibach HI. Contact urticaria to cosmetic and industrial dyes. Clin Exp Dermatol. 2011;36(1):1–5.

24. Rubegni P, Fimiani M, de Aloe G, Andreassi L. Lichenoid reaction to temporary tattoo. Contact Dermatitis. 2000;42(2):117–8.

25. Kheir A, Gaber I, Gafer S, Ahmed W. Life-threatening haemolysis induced by henna in a Sudanese child with glucose-6-phosphate dehydrogenase deficiency. East Mediterr Health J. 2017;23(1):28–30.

26. Raupp P, Hassan JA, Varughese M, Kristiansson B. Henna causes life threatening haemolysis in glucose-6-phosphate dehydrogenase deficiency. Arch Dis Child. 2001;85(5):411–2.

27. Sinha A, Goel L, Ranjan R, Gaba S, Kumar A. Atraumatic acute compartment syndrome of forearm following artificial mehndi (henna) dermatitis – a rare case report. J Clin Diagn Res. 2017;11(6):RD01–3.

28. Khine YY. Acute kidney injury following ingestion of henna leaf extract: a case report from Myanmar. Blood Purif. 2017;44(Suppl 1):41–5.

29. Guven SG. Dyspnea associated with henna stone: a rare cause of pediatric tracheotomy. Turk Arch Otorhinolaryngol. 2017;55(1):38–40.

30. Khanna N. Hand dermatitis in beauticians in India. Indian J Dermatol Venereol Leprol. 1997;63(3):157–61.

31. Lin LY, Chiou SC, Wang SH, Chi CC. Effects of facial threading on female skin texture: a prospective trial with physiological parameters and sense assessment. Evid Based Complement Alternat Med. 2019;2019:1535713.

32. Bloom MW, Carter EL. Bullous impetigo of the face after epilation by threading. Arch Dermatol. 2005;141(9):1174–5.

33. Abdel-Gawad MM, Abdel-Hamid IA, Wagner RF Jr. Khite: a non-Western technique for temporary hair removal. Int J Dermatol. 1997;36(3):217.

34. Halder S, Halder A. Verruca plana following eyebrow threading. Indian J Dermatol Venereol Leprol. 2009;75(2):196–7.

35. Kumar R, Zawar V. Threading warts: a beauty parlor dermatosis. J Cosmet Dermatol. 2007;6(4):279–82.

36. Sidharth S, Rahul A, Rashmi S. Cosmetic warts: pseudo-koebnerization of warts after cosmetic procedures for hair removal. J Clin Aesthet Dermatol. 2015;8(7):52–6.

37. Ghosh SK, Bandyopadhyay D. Molluscum contagiosum after eyebrow shaping: a beauty salon hazard. Clin Exp Dermatol. 2009;34(7):e339–40.

38. Verma SB. Eyebrow threading: a popular hair-removal procedure and its seldom-discussed complications. Clin Exp Dermatol. 2009;34(3):363–5.

39. Verma SB. Vitiligo koebnerized by eyebrow plucking by threading. J Cosmet Dermatol. 2002;1(4):214–5.

40. Litak J, Krunic AL, Antonijevic S, Pouryazdanparast P, Gerami P. Eyebrow epilation by threading: an increasingly popular

procedure with some less-popular outcomes--a comprehensive review. Dermatol Surg. 2011;37(7):1051–4.

41. Lilly E, Kundu RV. Dermatoses secondary to Asian cultural practices. Int J Dermatol. 2012;51(4):372–9; quiz 379–382.

42. Mehta SS, Reddy BS. Cosmetic dermatitis – current perspectives. Int J Dermatol. 2003;42(7):533–42.

43. Tewary M, Ahmed I. Bindi dermatitis to 'chandan' bindi. Contact Dermatitis. 2006;55(6):372–4.

44. Laxmisha C, Nath AK, Thappa DM. Bindi dermatitis due to thimerosal and gallate mix. J Eur Acad Dermatol Venereol. 2006;20(10):1370–2.

45. Nath AK, Thappa DM. Kumkum-induced dermatitis: an analysis of 46 cases. Clin Exp Dermatol. 2007;32(4):385–7.

46. Annabathula A, Priya S, Srinivas CR. Kumkum-induced allergic contact dermatitis: are we missing the actual culprit? Indian J Dermatol Venereol Leprol. 2018;84(2):153–6.

47. Kozuka I, Goh CL, Doi T, Yioshikawa K. Sudan I as a cause of pigmented contact dermatitis in "kumkum" (an Indian cosmetic). Ann Acad Med Singap. 1988;17(4):492–4.

48. Kumar JV, Moideen R, Murugesh SB. Contactants in 'KumKum' dermatitis. Indian J Dermatol Venereol Leprol. 1996;62(4):220–1.

49. Pandhi D, Vij A, Singal A. Contact depigmentation induced by propyl gallate. Clin Exp Dermatol. 2011;36(4):366–8.

50. Baxter KF, Wilkinson SM. Contact dermatitis from a nickel-containing bindi. Contact Dermatitis. 2002;47(1):55.

51. Dwyer CM, Forsyth A. Allergic contact dermatitis from bindi. Contact Dermatitis. 1994;30(3):174.

52. Bajaj AK, Gupta SC, Chatterjee AK. Contact depigmentation from free para-tertiary-butylphenol in bindi adhesive. Contact Dermatitis. 1990;22(2):99–102.

53. Chatierjee A, Bajaj AK, Gupta SC. Identification of a contact depigmenting agent in Indian bindi. Natl Med J India. 1991;4(3):113–5.

54. Mathur AK, Srivastava AK, Singh A, Gupta BN. Contact depigmentation by adhesive material of bindi. Contact Dermatitis. 1991;24(4):310–1.

55. Pandhi RK, Kumar AS. Contact leukoderma due to 'Bindi' and footwear. Dermatologica. 1985;170(5):260–2.

56. Bajaj AK, Govil DC, Bajaj S. Bindi depigmentation. Arch Dermatol. 1983;119(8):629.

57. Goyal S, Sajid N, Husain S. Contact dermatitis due to local cosmetics: a study from Northern India. Indian J Dermatol. 2019;64(6):461–4.

58. Singh P, Singh J, Agarwal US, Bhargava RK. Contact vitiligo: etiology and treatment. Indian J Dermatol Venereol Leprol. 2003;69(1):27–9.

59. Goh CL, Kozuka T. Pigmented contact dermatitis from 'kumkum'. Clin Exp Dermatol. 1986;11(6):603–6.

60. Mishra G, Rathi S, Mulani J. Bindi tuberculosis – lupus vulgaris associated with bindi use: a case report. J Clin Diagn Res. 2015;9(5):Od04–5.

61. Kumar AS, Pandhi RK, Bhutani LK. Bindi dermatoses. Int J Dermatol. 1986;25(7):434–5.

62. Ramesh V. Foreign-body granuloma on the forehead: reaction to bindi. Arch Dermatol. 1991;127(3):424.

63. Verma SB. Dermatological signs in South Asian women induced by sari and petticoat drawstrings. Clin Exp Dermatol. 2010;35(5):459–61.

64. Kumara L, Rangaraj M, Karthikeyan K. Drawstring lichen planus: a unique case of Koebnerization. Indian Dermatol Online J. 2016;7(3):201–2.

65. Eapen BR, Shabana S, Anandan S. Waist dermatoses in Indian women wearing saree. Indian J Dermatol Venereol Leprol. 2003;69(2):88–9.

66. Stirn A. Body piercing: medical consequences and psychological motivations. Lancet. 2003;361(9364):1205–15.

67. Meltzer DI. Complications of body piercing. Am Fam Physician. 2005;72(10):2029–34.

68. Ladizinski B, Nutan FN, Lee KC. Nose piercing: historical significance and potential consequences. JAMA Dermatol. 2013;149(2):142.

69. Kumar Ghosh S, Bandyopadhyay D. Granuloma pyogenicum as a complication of decorative nose piercing: report of eight cases from eastern India. J Cutan Med Surg. 2012;16(3):197–200.

70. Kluger N, Gaudy-Marquestre C, Monestier S, Hesse S, Jacques Grob J, Aleth RM. Persistent telangiectatic erythema following nostril piercing. Int J Dermatol. 2014;53(2):e149–51.

71. Khundkar R, Wilson PA. Basal cell carcinoma at the site of a nasal piercing. J Plast Reconstr Aesthet Surg. 2009;62(4):557–8.

72. Roman J. African scarification. JAMA Dermatol. 2016;152(12):1353.

73. Tsiba JB, Mabiala-Babela JR, Lenga LI, et al. Scarification in children hospitalized in Congo. Med Trop (Mars). 2011;71(5):509–10.

74. Mammen L, Norton SA. Facial scarification and tattooing on Santa Catalina Island (Solomon Islands). Cutis. 1997;60(4):197–8.

75. Dunyo SK, Ahorlu CK, Simonsen PE. Scarification as a risk factor for rapid progression of filarial elephantiasis. Trans R Soc Trop Med Hyg. 1997;91(4):446.

76. Hrdy DB. Cultural practices contributing to the transmission of human immunodeficiency virus in Africa. Rev Infect Dis. 1987;9(6):1109–19.

77. Ayoola EA. Infectious diseases in Africa. Infection. 1987;15(3):153–9.

78. Alabi GO, George AO. Cutaneous sarcoidosis and tribal scarifications in West Africa. Int J Dermatol. 1989;28(1):29–31.

79. Kaatz M, Elsner P, Bauer A. Body-modifying concepts and dermatologic problems: tattooing and piercing. Clin Dermatol. 2008;26(1):35–44.

80. Babatunde OP, Oyeronke AE. Scarification practice and scar complications among the Nigerian Yorubas. Indian J Dermatol Venereol Leprol. 2010;76(5):571–2.

81. Kamagaju L, Morandini R, Gahongayire F, et al. Survey on skin-lightening practices and cosmetics in Kigali, Rwanda. Int J Dermatol. 2016;55(1):45–51.

82. Petit A, Cohen-Ludmann C, Clevenbergh P, Bergmann JF, Dubertret L. Skin lightening and its complications among African people living in Paris. J Am Acad Dermatol. 2006;55(5):873–8.

83. Ho YB, Abdullah NH, Hamsan H, Tan ESS. Mercury contamination in facial skin lightening creams and its health risks to user. Regul Toxicol Pharmacol. 2017;88:72–6.

84. Cristaudo A, D'Ilio S, Gallinella B, et al. Use of potentially harmful skin-lightening products among immigrant women in Rome, Italy: a pilot study. Dermatology. 2013;226(3):200–6.

85. Hollick EJ, Igwe C, Papamichael E, et al. Corneal and scleral problems caused by skin-lightening creams. Cornea. 2019;38(10):1332–5.

86. Dlova NC, Hamed SH, Tsoka-Gwegweni J, Grobler A. Skin lightening practices: an epidemiological study of South African women of African and Indian ancestries. Br J Dermatol. 2015;173(Suppl 2):2–9.

87. Draelos ZD. Skin lightening preparations and the hydroquinone controversy. Dermatol Ther. 2007;20(5):308–13.
88. Oliveira A, Amaro C, Cardoso J. Allergic contact dermatitis caused by sodium metabisulphite in a cosmetic bleaching cream. Australas J Dermatol. 2015;56(2):144–5.
89. Garcia-Gavin J, Gonzalez-Vilas D, Fernandez-Redondo V, Toribio J. Pigmented contact dermatitis due to kojic acid. A paradoxical side effect of a skin lightener. Contact Dermatitis. 2010;62(1):63–4.
90. Suzuki K, Yagami A, Matsunaga K. Allergic contact dermatitis caused by a skin-lightening agent, 5,5′-dipropylbiphenyl-2,2′-diol. Contact Dermatitis. 2012;66(1):51–2.
91. Gohara M, Yagami A, Suzuki K, et al. Allergic contact dermatitis caused by phenylethyl resorcinol [4-(1-phenylethyl)-1,3-benzenediol], a skin-lightening agent in cosmetics. Contact Dermatitis. 2013;69(5):319–20.
92. Mamodaly M, Dereure O, Raison-Peyron N. A new case of allergic contact dermatitis caused by 3-o-ethyl ascorbic acid in facial antiageing cosmetics. Contact Dermatitis. 2019;81(4):315–6.
93. Dilokthornsakul W, Dhippayom T, Dilokthornsakul P. The clinical effect of glutathione on skin color and other related skin conditions: a systematic review. J Cosmet Dermatol. 2019;18(3):728–37.
94. Hamann CR, Boonchai W, Wen L, et al. Spectrometric analysis of mercury content in 549 skin-lightening products: is mercury toxicity a hidden global health hazard? J Am Acad Dermatol. 2014;70(2):281–287.e283.
95. Iwegbue CM, Bassey FI, Tesi GO, Onyeloni SO, Obi G, Martincigh BS. Safety evaluation of metal exposure from commonly used moisturizing and skin-lightening creams in Nigeria. Regul Toxicol Pharmacol. 2015;71(3):484–90.
96. del Giudice P, Yves P. The widespread use of skin lightening creams in Senegal: a persistent public health problem in West Africa. Int J Dermatol. 2002;41(2):69–72.
97. Tatebayashi M, Oiso N, Wada T, Suzuki K, Matsunaga K, Kawada A. Possible allergic contact dermatitis with reticulate postinflammatory pigmentation caused by hydroquinone. J Dermatol. 2014;41(7):669–70.
98. Numata T, Kobayashi Y, Ito T, Harada K, Tsuboi R, Okubo Y. Two cases of allergic contact dermatitis due to skin-whitening cosmetics. Allergol Int. 2015;64(2):194–5.

99. Numata T, Tobita R, Tsuboi R, Okubo Y. Contact dermatitis caused by arbutin contained in skin-whitening cosmetics. Contact Dermatitis. 2016;75(3):187–8.

100. Lecamwasam KL, Lim TM, Fuller LC. Tinea incognito caused by skin-lightening products. J Eur Acad Dermatol Venereol. 2016;30(3):480–1.

101. Yagami A, Suzuki K, Sano A, et al. Rhododendrol-induced leukoderma accompanied by allergic contact dermatitis caused by a non-rhododendrol skin-lightening agent, 5,5′-dipropylbiphenyl-2,2′-diol. J Dermatol. 2015;42(7):739–40.

102. Faye O, Dicko AA, Berthe S, et al. Squamous cell carcinoma associated with use of skin-lightening cream. Ann Dermatol Venereol. 2018;145(2):100–3.

103. Totri CR, Diaz L, Matiz C, Krakowski AC. A 15-year-old girl with painful, peeling skin. Pediatr Ann. 2015;44(5):195–7.

104. Olumide YM, Akinkugbe AO, Altraide D, et al. Complications of chronic use of skin lightening cosmetics. Int J Dermatol. 2008;47(4):344–53.

105. Scheinfeld N. Tattoos and religion. Clin Dermatol. 2007;25(4):362–6.

106. Telang GH, Ditre CM. Blue gingiva, an unusual oral pigmentation resulting from gingival tattoo. J Am Acad Dermatol. 1994;30(1):125–6.

107. Islam PS, Chang C, Selmi C, et al. Medical complications of tattoos: a comprehensive review. Clin Rev Allergy Immunol. 2016;50(2):273–86.

108. Kluger N. Cutaneous and systemic complications associated with tattooing. Presse Med. 2016;45(6 Pt 1):567–76.

Chapter 3
Cultural Hair-Related Dermatoses

Casey C. Bunge and Roopal V. Kundu

Ethnic hair has distinct biology. The tight curls and kinks often seen in Black hair impact sebum transport as well as introduce frictional forces [1]. Such biological factors, in addition to cultural perceptions of beauty, have inspired the development of several cultural hair practices designed to beautify ethnic hair or make it easier to manage and style. These include use of hair oils, hair restructuring techniques, and hair styling techniques.

However, cultural hair care practices can have side effects, including allergic contact dermatitis (ACD) and alopecia. It is therefore important that the practicing dermatologist be aware of such practices and their associated complications. Understanding patients' cultural backgrounds and habits will also enable more informed counseling, leading to a more supportive and fulfilling patient-physician relationship [2].

C. C. Bunge · R. V. Kundu (✉)
Department of Dermatology, Northwestern University Feinberg School of Medicine, Chicago, IL, USA
e-mail: roopal.kundu@nm.org

© The Author(s) 2021
N. A. Vashi (ed.), *Cultural Practices and Dermatoses*,
https://doi.org/10.1007/978-3-030-68992-6_3

51

Cultural and Psychosocial Significance

Hair care is a particularly important aspect of cultural practice due to the relationship between hair appearance and measures of quality of life, self-esteem, and self-confidence [3]. One survey of 58 women with alopecia revealed that 75% had experienced loss of confidence, and 88% changed their daily routine as a result of their hair loss [4]. Another survey used the Dermatology Life Quality Index to find that patients with hair loss experienced significant changes in self-confidence, self-esteem, and self-consciousness – and that 40% were unhappy with their treatment by a physician [5]. Further, narrative accounts have illustrated the importance of hair treatments in establishing personal and cultural identity, particularly among Black Americans [6, 7]. These are important considerations to bear in mind when discussing hair care practices with patients of color.

Hair Oil Dermatoses

Hair oils provide external nutrition with the purported benefits of softening, shining, and promoting hair growth, along with preventing hair loss [8]. These oils can be added to shampoos and conditioners, or they can be applied directly by massaging into the scalp and then rubbed over the length of the hair.

The most used oils are carrier oils such as castor or coconut [9]. Similar to natural sebum, carriers typically consist of hydrophobic compounds including free fatty acids, triglycerides, phenols, sterols, and squalene [10]. Other potential components are amino acids, minerals, vitamin E, and other antioxidants [11]. Additionally, some users mix the base oil with herbal elements or an essential oil prior to application [12, 13]. This can provide additional vitamins and minerals, amino acids, and fatty acids to the hair shaft. Examples include lavender and bhringraj oil [8].

Use of hair oil is common among populations with curly hair, including Asian Indians, Hispanics, Africans, and Black Americans. This may be because the geometry of curly hair leaves it less lubricated by natural sebum, rendering such hair more prone to breakage and frizz. Furthermore, hair oils are important for reducing friction and resultant damage during the styling and chemical treatment of ethnic hair [1].

Along with the noted benefits, application of hair oils may have other dermatologic effects. Some products are known sensitizers leading to allergic contact dermatitis, while others may exacerbate seborrheic dermatitis. Interestingly, some oils have demonstrated anti-microbial effects and may confer protection against tinea capitis. Commonly used hair oils are summarized in Table 3.1.

Carrier Oils

Almond Oil

Almond oil is a commonly used hair oil in India [8]. It is composed of up to 80% oleic acid and also contains linoleic and palmitic acids [14].

There is one case report of an atopic child who developed contact dermatitis to almond oil. This occurred after applying the oil focally to areas of atopic dermatitis for 2 months, and without ingesting the oil [15].

Amla Oil

A 1992 survey found that amla oil was one of the most commonly used hair oils in India [16]. It contains predominantly unsaturated long-chain fatty acids.

The oil has demonstrated anti-fungal activity, capable of inhibiting growth of *Microsporum canis*, *M. gypseum,* and

TABLE 3.1 Summary of commonly used hair oils

Oil	Sensitizer	Notes
Almond	No	Commonly used in India, 1 report of ACD, in an atopic child
Amla	No	Commonly used in india, Demonstrates broad anti-fungal activity
Argan	Yes	Reports of ACD, 1 report of anaphylaxis
Castor	Yes	1 report of acute hair felting associated with castor oil use
Coconut	No	Derivatives, such as cocamidopropyl betaine, may act as sensitizers and irritants, demonstrates anti-microbial activity
Jojoba	Yes	Reports of ACD
Mustard	Yes	Reports of ACD
Olive	Yes	High oleic acid content may exacerbate seborrheic dermatitis; olive oil should be avoided in treatment of cradle cap
Shea Butter	No	May increase friction during combing, leading to hair breakage
Lavender	Yes	Ingredients become oxidized over time. When patch testing, it is recommended to use the patient's product
Tea tree	Yes	Often applied as an anti-inflammatory. Ingredients become oxidized over time.
E. alba	No	Commonly used in Ayurvedic tradition

Trychophyton rubrum. This antimicrobial property is thought to be a result of its high concentration of unsaturated fatty acids, which are more toxic to fungi than saturated molecules [16]. No reports of allergic contact dermatitis have been published thus far.

Argan Oil

Recently developed, argan oil has become increasingly popular over the last two decades as both a moisturizing hair oil and as a skin treatment. It is primarily composed of the unsaturated long chain fatty acids oleic and linoleic. Its high tocopherol content renders it an excellent antioxidant, driving some of its popularity [17].

Several cases of argan oil-associated allergic contact dermatitis have been reported [18]. One case developed in a woman using argan oil as a hair product, presenting with pruritus, drainage, and an eczematous dermatitis on the scalp [19]. One man was reported to experience rhinitis and conjunctivitis upon smelling argan oil, and after ingesting it, developed anaphylaxis [20].

Castor Oil

Castor oil is often used during hair treatments to soften and moisturize the hair [9]. It can also be found in shampoos, hair dyes, and various hygiene products [21]. As an oil, it is frequently used by those with thinning hair in efforts to stimulate hair regrowth. However, while the thickness of castor oil makes hair appear fuller, there is no published evidence that it induces regrowth [21].

The main ingredient of castor oil is ricinoleic acid, a known sensitizer which can lead to the development of allergic contact dermatitis [9]. Castor oil associated ACD has been reported with use of multiple hygiene and cosmetic products including lipsticks [22, 23], makeup removers [24], and deodorants [25].

In one patient, one time use of castor oil triggered acute hair felting. After application with the viscous oil and washing with warm water, the patient's hair tangled and sealed into a hard mass "resembling a bird's nest." This was associated with pain at the hair roots as well as emotional distress. Due to the irreversibility of hair felting, the only treatment available was cutting the matted hair [26].

Coconut Oil

Coconut oil is commonly used by Black Americans and Asian Indians. A 1992 survey found that it was the most used hair oil among Asian Indian women and the second most used by Asian Indian men [16]. Its primary component is lauric acid [16], a relatively small, linear molecule thought to penetrate the hair shaft and bind hair proteins with high affinity. This may be why use of coconut oil has been associated with increased retention of hair protein [27].

Additionally, coconut oil has demonstrated anti-microbial activity. It is toxic to the dermatophyte *Trichophyton mentagrophtes*, completely inhibiting all fungal growth at concentrations as low as 5 parts per 1000 [16]. This anti-fungal effect appears to be specific, as the oil exhibited significantly weaker effects on other dermatophytes.

Coconut oil has also been shown to reduce *Staphylococcus aureus* colonization in patients with atopic dermatitis (AD). In a double-blind controlled trial, 52 AD subjects were randomized to receive either coconut oil or olive oil [28]. Subjects were instructed to apply 5 mL of oil for several seconds twice a day. At the end of the trial, the number of subjects infected with *S. aureus* decreased by 95% relative to baseline among those using coconut oil, compared to a 50% reduction seen in those using olive oil.

The anti-microbial properties of coconut oil are attributed to the relatively small size of its fatty acids. These molecules are thought to diffuse into and disrupt the bacterial cell membrane as well as inhibit crucial metabolic enzymes. A laboratory study showed that monoglycerides of medium chain fatty acids exhibited bactericidal effects on gram-positive cocci [29], concordant with the clinical results described above.

A report by the Cosmetics Ingredients Expert Review Panel found that coconut oil itself is a non-irritant and a non-sensitizer [30]. However, coconut oil derivatives have been shown to elicit allergic responses. One such derivative, cocamidopropyl betaine, is a synthetic detergent used in some shampoos as well as other hygiene products including soaps and makeup removers [31]. There have been many reports in the literature of allergic contact dermatitis resulting from use of products containing the compound. While ACD is more common, cocamidopropyl betaine-associated irritant contact dermatitis has also been reported [32]. Follow-up studies have demonstrated that the true sensitizing allergen is dimethylaminopropylamine, an impurity left over from cocamidoproyl betaine synthesis [33]. Persons exposed to cocamidopropyl betaine-containing products are thus at risk of developing ACD or, less commonly, ICD.

One case was reported of a 6-month-old boy who developed persistent pneumonia secondary to coconut oil aspiration [34]. The child was feeding on hair oil at home and quickly developed cough and respiratory distress. Imaging and biopsy revealed signs of lipoid pneumonia, a type of aspiration pneumonia associated with inhalation of fatty substances. The case resolved after 8 weeks of supplemental oxygen and 3 months of oral steroids. This case highlights the importance of educating patients on potential health hazards facing young children with easy access to hair oils.

Jojoba Oil

Jojoba oil is an increasingly popular product among Black Americans [9]. It has a relatively large concentration of wax esters, similar to natural sebum, resulting in its advertisement as a 'natural' component of various hair and skin cosmetic products. Interestingly, jojoba oil has demonstrated anti-inflammatory properties in various animal models, including the reduction of edema after skin insult [35]. An in vitro study of effects on human keratinocytes and fibroblasts revealed acceleration of wound closure and stimulation of collagen I synthesis upon application of jojoba oil. Due to these effects, the authors postulated that the oil may find use in clinical settings [36].

Jojoba oil has been associated with the development of allergic contact dermatitis. One study found that five individuals suspected of jojoba oil sensitivity developed erythema with or without vesicles upon patch testing. A sixth had a negative reaction to skin patch testing, but repeatedly demonstrated contact dermatitis on the scalp after application of pure jojoba oil to the hair [37]. A further case was reported of a woman who developed erythematous pomphoid lesions diffusely over the body after application of a body cream containing jojoba oil, with sensitivity confirmed via patch testing [38]. Another woman developed dermatitis and pruritus on her face after several years of applying a moisturizing cream containing jojoba oil, and subsequently demonstrated a positive reaction to jojoba seed powder on patch test [39].

Mustard Oil

Mustard oil is a commonly used hair oil, and a 1992 survey indicated that it was the most used oil among Asian Indian men at the time [16]. Chemically, it is composed primarily of fatty acid chains longer than 20 carbons.

In two patients, use of mustard oil triggered contact dermatitis over the hands, face, and neck, with hypersensitivity to mustard oil confirmed via patch testing [40]. In one patient, mustard oil contact dermatitis presented with pityriasis-rosea like eruptions [41]. Hypersensitivity to the oil has been attributed to a specific component, allyl isothiocyanate [17].

Olive Oil

Olive oil is a popular hair oil among Black Americans. Primarily comprised of oleic acid, it is often used to treat dandruff and promote hair growth [9].

Olive oil is commonly used to treat infantile seborrheic dermatitis, or 'cradle cap' [42]. It may be ill-suited for this indication, however, owing to its high oleic acid content and saturated lipid profile. Application of pure oleic acid to the scalp has been shown to trigger desquamation and scale, even in the absence of *Malassezia spp.* [43]. Furthermore, *Malassezia* is known to thrive on the saturated fatty acid content of olive oil as a source of nutrients [43]. As such, it is recommended that olive oil, and other organic oils, be avoided in the treatment of seborrheic dermatitis [42].

Shea Butter

Unique among the frequently used hair oils, shea butter is thick and solid at room temperature. It is a fat composed primarily of oleic and stearic acid. Common uses include skin moisturizing and hair care, and it is a popular choice among people of African descent [9]. As a hair product, shea butter finds use as a thick moisturizer and in the management of highly textured hair.

The use of shea butter in hair is not well-studied. Various formulations have been tested on human skin, with no evidence of irritation or sensitization reactions [30]. However, caution is warranted, as thick butters similar to shea butter have been shown to increase friction during combing. This can induce mechanical damage such as split ends [9].

Herbs and Essential Oils

Lavender Oil

The essential oil of lavender is obtained from the flowering tops of the evergreen dwarf shrub *Lavandula angustifolia Mill* [44]. Its primary components are linalyl acetate and linalool, oxidized derivatives of terpenes. A common fragrant used in many foods, cosmetics, and herbal medicine products, lavender oil is also touted as an aromatherapeutic anxiolytic. When used as a hair oil, it is often mixed with a carrier oil prior to application.

Several cases of lavender oil-associated contact dermatitis have been reported [45]. One patient using aroma lamps developed an allergic airborne contact dermatitis on the head, neck, and hands after becoming sensitized to lavender and other essential oils in aromatherapy products [46]. One patient developed a vulvovaginitis exacerbated by contact dermatitis from a product containing tea tree and lavender oil [47]. There have also been reports of photocontact allergy to lavender oil as well, particularly to products containing ketoprofen as a vehicle [48, 49]. Further, occupational dermatitis has been noted among a hairdresser [50] and several massage therapists [51–53] using lavender oil.

Sensitivity to lavender oil is due to oxidation of its primary components upon exposure to air. Linalyl acetate and linalool themselves are very weak allergens [45]. However, they are readily autoxidized, creating hydroperoxides [54, 55]. These hydroperoxides are potent contact allergens to which hypersensitivity develops in lavender oil ACD [56].

Tea Tree

Tea tree oil is extracted from the tea tree *Melaleuca alternifolia* native to Australia [57]. Primary constituents include various terpene alcohols, such as terpinen-4-ol and γ-terpinene [58]. It is commonly used as a hair oil by Black Americans [9], and it can also be found in cleaning and cosmetic products [57].

The purported benefits of tea tree oil are manifold, including anti-fungal activity. One randomized controlled trial of 126 subjects with seborrheic dermatitis tested the activity of 5% tea tree oil shampoo. Relative to placebo, the results demonstrated significant improvement in the quadrant-area-severity score as well as itchiness and greasiness, with no reported adverse effects [59]. An RCT of 117 subjects suggested that a 100% tea tree oil cream was as effective as 1% clotrimazole in resolving culture-positive onychomycosis in 6 months (60% vs 61%, p > .05, [60]). In vitro studies suggest broad anti-fungal activity [61] by way of disrupting membrane function [62] and respiration [63]. Tea tree oil has also shown broad-spectrum bactericidal activity by similar mechanisms [63], with concentrations as low as 0.625% demonstrated to be lethal to MRSA in vitro [64]. Other studies indicate anti-HSV [65] and anti-protozoal [66] activity as well.

Tea tree oil may also have anti-inflammatory properties. It was shown to significantly reduce histamine-induced wheal formation in one study of 27 subjects [67]. A further study recreated these findings and identified terpinen-4-ol as the causative agent [68].

However, many reports have implicated tea tree oil in allergic contact dermatitis. In roughly two-thirds of these cases, pure tea tree oil was applied to previously damaged skin for therapeutic purposes, such as treatment of acne, eczema, wounds, warts, and fungal infections [57]. Occupational contact dermatitis was noted in six patients. Other reports of ACD involved products containing tea tree oil in concentrations of 2% or greater.

As with lavender oil, tea tree oil ingredients become oxidized upon prolonged or repeated exposure to air [57]. The terpene alcohols can react to form peroxides and epoxides such as ascaridole [69], and later 1,2,4-trihydroxymenthane [70]. Patients with tea tree oil contact dermatitis have positive reactions to ascaridole 84% (51/61) of the time, and to 1,2,4-trihydroxymenthane 62% (43/69) of the time, highlighting their importance in the development of ACD [57]. Because the formulation can change with age and oxidation, it is recommended to patch test using patients' own products containing tea tree oil [9].

Eclipta Alba

Eclipta alba Hassk. (Asteraceae) is an herb native to Bangladesh [71]. Several chemical components have been reported, including alkaloids, sterols, and alkanes [72]. The herb has found many uses in Asian Indian Ayurvedic tradition, including as an anti-inflammatory, a hepatoprotective, and an antimicrobial agent. When used for hair growth, oil is extracted from the plant – often referred to as bhrinraj oil – and is applied to the hair [72]. No hypersensitivity reactions to *Eclipta alba* have been reported thus far.

Dermatoses

Seborrheic Dermatitis

Organic hair oils – especially those with high oleic acid content such as olive oil or sesame oil – may trigger seborrheic dermatitis. Application of pure oleic acid to the scalp has been shown to trigger desquamation and flaking, even in the absence of *Malassezia spp.* [43]. Further, *Malassezia* is known to subsist on saturated fatty acids as a source of nutrients [43]. Hair oils may thus promote the growth of *Malassezia* and even directly cause desquamation. As such, it is recommended that olive oil and other organic oils be avoided in the treatment of seborrheic dermatitis and cradle cap [42].

Mudichood

Mudichood, translating to "heat of the hair," is a rare dermatosis that typically presents in South Indian women during the summer months. It is a follicular reaction to prolonged contact between comedogenic hair oils and the skin of the neck and upper back, especially in the context of excessive heat and humidity [8]. It presents as a lichenoid dermatitis with well-defined pruritic papules that may exhibit Koebner's phenomenon [73].

Dermoscopy findings were recently described [74] as three zones centered around a hypopigmented hair follicle. From central to peripheral, the zones include (1) a hypopigmented zone within the papule; (2) a relatively hyperpigmented zone within the papule; and (3) a thin keratinous and slightly erythematous rim. On pathology, papules demonstrate hyperkeratosis, focal parakeratosis, acanthosis, and dermal edema with dilated capillaries. The condition can be treated with topical steroids with discontinuation of the culprit hair oils [75, 76].

Hair Restructuring Techniques

Hair restructuring techniques are commonly used to make ethnic hair more manageable by reducing volume, kinks, and frizz [77]. They are common among populations with thick, curly or kinky hair, such as Asian Indians, Black Americans, and Hispanics. The benefits are primarily practical and aesthetic. In one survey of women using chemical hair relaxers, the main reasons expressed for their use included making hair more manageable and easy to style as well as yielding a more "beautiful" appearance [78]. Discussed below are several hair restructuring methods that are available depending on convenience and desired hairstyle.

Thermal Straightening (Hot Combing)

Hot combing was among the first methods used to restructure hair. A comb is heated to 150–500 °F and then pulled through the length of the hair, allowing the heat to disrupt disulfide bonds in keratin [79]. If water is avoided, restructuring via this technique typically allows for 1–2 weeks of straightening before perspiration and humidity cause the hair to regain its natural shape [3].

Thermal straightening carries several risks related to heat exposure [3]. Accidental application of the hot comb to the skin can result in moderate to severe burns. Even with careful use, high heat can cause severe damage to the hair shaft as well, resulting in hair weakening or breakage. Hot comb use has also been associated with development of central centrifugal cicatricial alopecia (CCCA) [80].

Chemical Hair Relaxers

Relaxers are chemicals straighteners and present a more modern method of restructuring hair [1]. These products use various alkaline salts: lye formulations use sodium hydroxide, while no-lye compositions contain calcium hydroxide/guanidine hydroxide or ammonium thioglycolate. The high pH in relaxers causes the hair to swell which allows hydroxide molecules to further penetrate and disrupt disulfide bonds in keratin, resulting in straightened hair [81]. Chemical relaxers have found popularity as they offer more permanent control of kinks and curls – they need only be reapplied when new hair has grown long enough to be treated [3]. A survey of 90 Asian Indian women reported that 'beautification' and 'ease of management' were the greatest perceived benefits of the treatment [82].

Chemical relaxer use has been associated with dermatoses in multiple patients. A survey of 90 Asian Indian women found that frizzy hair (67%), dandruff (60%), and hair loss (47%) were the most common side effects of hair relaxer use, followed by reports of thinning and weakened hair (40%), greying of hair (22%), and split ends (17%) [82]. A case series reported five patients each of whom developed an alopecia associated with hair relaxer use. Pathology was characterized by concentric perifollicular scarring and premature desquamation of the inner root sheath [83]. Another woman developed a hair relaxer-mediated irritant contact dermatitis that was later complicated by *Staphylococcus Aureus* infection [84].

Systemic symptoms are possible as well. An analysis of the Black Women's Health Study found a correlation between hair relaxer use and uterine leiomyomata confirmed by ultrasound (incidence rate ratio = 1.17; 95% CI: 1.06–1.30). Significant trends were noted for frequency of use ($p < 0.001$), duration of use ($p = 0.015$), and number of burns ($p < 0.001$) [85]. Finally, use of hair relaxers triggered Stevens-Johnson syndrome in one patient, who recovered with supportive treatment and oral prednisolone [86].

Brazilian Keratin Treatments

Brazilian keratin hair treatments (BKT) have become increasingly popular since the early 2000s [87]. Early formulations of these products contained large concentrations of formaldehyde, while more recent versions are marketed as "formaldehyde-free" [1]. However, these newer products contain formaldehyde-producing agents such as glyoxylic acid or methylene glycol, and may still be dangerous. One study tested seven brands of BKT marketed in South Africa and found that six contained formaldehyde concentrations greater than the maximum safe concentration set by the US Cosmetic Ingredient Review Expert Panel (< 0.2%) [88]. Indeed, the range for those six products was found to be 0.96–1.4%, five times higher than the recommended level. Five of the six products were marketed as 'formaldehyde-free.'

Mechanistically, in BKT, water disrupts hydrogen bonds in keratin while formaldehyde crosslinks proteins. One study revealed that formaldehyde can crosslink the amino acids arginine, lysine, tyrosine, histidine, glutamine, and asparagine in keratin [89] to exert its effect. The result is a smooth and shiny appearance that cannot be obtained through other methods [1]. Brazil keratin treatments are also compatible with bleached or dyed hair as well as other hair restructuring techniques, contributing to their popularity [87].

BKT carries health risks associated with formaldehyde exposure [1]. Eye irritation and burning of the throat can occur during exposure to concentrations greater than 0.1 part per million [90]. One study showed that during application of BKT, airborne concentrations of formaldehyde can reach 0.5 ppm; during blow-drying, levels can reach 3.5 ppm [91]. Further, a case series reported seven patients who developed eczema-like erythematous pustules and psoriasiform scaling on the scalp following BKT [92]. Contact allergen testing to formaldehyde was negative for all seven patients. Four patients were biopsied, and common findings included orthokeratosis, parakeratosis, hypogranulosis, psoriasiform acanthosis, and lymphocytic infiltrate. The authors considered this consistent with a drug reaction, similar to anti-TNFα scalp alopecia. A case of BKT-associated allergic contact dermatitis has also been reported, presenting as oozing eczema of the scalp, forehead, and neck and prominent eyelid edema [93]. Patch testing confirmed hypersensitivity to formaldehyde, which comprised 2.84% of the BKT product used. The patient's condition improved with 1 week of oral methylprednisolone.

Hair Styling Techniques and Associated Alopecias

Hair Styling Techniques

Braids

Braiding is a common hair styling technique used by men and women of many ethnic backgrounds [77]. It involves interweaving three or more strands of hair to create a textured appearance. Cornrows – a tight braid worn just atop the scalp – are a variation frequently worn by Black men and women [3]. Braids are often maintained for long periods of time for several reasons, including the time and financial investment involved with the styling choice [94].

Braids – especially the tight forms commonly worn by Black men and women – can produce traction and tension leading to hair damage [95]. In one study of Black American women, braided hair styles were found to be associated with non-scarring and scarring alopecia [94]. It is believed that long-term maintenance of braids, resulting in prolonged traction, may cause chronic folliculitis and ultimately scarring.

Excessive traction produced by braided hairstyles was implicated in scalp cutaneous necrosis in two patients. One was a 41-year-old woman who noted development of swelling and tenderness soon after a tight braid. After a couple days, this gave way to full-thickness skin ulceration of a roughly

10 cm × 7 cm area on the parietal scalp [96]. Another, an 18-year-old woman with a history of sickle cell trait, experienced 3 weeks of foul smelling discharge from the scalp before presenting with a 10 cm × 20 cm necrotic plaque [97]. The pathogenesis of this severe complication is unclear, but excessive traction and skin ischemia are hypothesized to play a role [96].

There have also been two case reports of subgaleal hematomas developing shortly after hair braiding. One patient was a 17-year-old boy with von Willebrand Disease who had had no complications after multiple previous braids [98]. However, a few days after a new braided hairstyle, he developed progressive swelling and pain over the frontal scalp. He presented to the emergency department where 340 cc of sanguineous fluid was aspirated; 3 days later, he returned to the ED with reaccumulation of fluid. Head CT revealed the subgaleal hematoma. A second patient was an 8-year-old girl who had her hair braided into cornrows [99]. Within a day of the braiding she complained of headache and scalp pain which progressed for the next 10 days before presenting to the emergency department. The patient was deemed hemodynamically stable and discharged without intervention, and the hematoma resolved 5.5 weeks later. Such braid-induced subgaleal hematomas may be more likely to occur in children; according to one report, children have a more vascular subaponeurotic space along with a thinner scalp relative to adults [100].

Weaves

Black American women often wear hair extensions, or weaves, that provide length, texture, and style. Extensions may be synthetic or made of human hair, and they can be either sewn onto cornrows or applied via bonding glue [101].

Weaves add weight to the hair which can result in excessive tension. As such, traction folliculitis and traction alopecia have been associated with weave use [102]. Also, as with braids, the increased traction may lead to CCCA. One study found that CCCA patients were more likely to endorse previous use of hair weaves than non-CCCA patients. Weave-wearers who developed CCCA were also more likely to report clinical symptoms of "tender scalp" and "uncomfortable pulling" [95].

When glues are used to apply weaves, users may develop allergic reactions to the latex in bonding adhesives. One case report described a patient's systemic anaphylaxis after their second exposure to bonding glue. This was found to be a result of latex allergy. The patient improved after immediate removal of the glue and taking 25 mg of diphenhydramine [103].

Alopecias

Traction Alopecia

Traction alopecia begins as a noncicatricial hair loss resulting from excessive prolonged tension on the hair. Among Black women and girls, tight braids (e.g. cornrows) and weaves have been implicated [102, 104, 105]. The condition has also been seen in the hair and beards of Sikh boys and men who style their hair very tightly [106, 107]. It has been noted in Hispanic patients as well, particularly affecting those with long, thick hair who wear tight ponytails [108].

Traction alopecia typically presents on the frontal and parietal scalp, with pruritus and erythema as the first signs of pathology [109]. A hyperkeratosis may develop as well. As the disease progresses, follicles involute and the hair becomes shorter and thinner. Prolonged traction can also produce an irritating folliculitis. Finally, if not resolved, an irreversible scarring alopecia can develop [95].

It is important to identify traction alopecia early in its progression, especially among children, given the potential for permanent damage. If identified, the causative hair styling method must be immediately discontinued. In mild cases, full hair growth can recur within a few months of wearing the hair more loosely [107]. Should folliculitis develop, use of oral and topical antibiotics are indicated. Inflammation can be treated with topical corticosteroids [101]. 2% topical minoxidil has been reported as an effective treatment in recovering hair loss caused by traction alopecia [83]. Severe cases of traction alopecia may benefit from surgical correction [110].

Central Centrifugal Cicatricial Alopecia (CCCA)

Central centrifugal cicatricial alopecia is the most common scarring alopecia among Black Americans [111]. The condition has been associated with braids [94] and various forms of extensions, including sewn-in and glued-on weaves [95]. Its previous title, "hot comb alopecia," reveals an additional association with heat damage. Indeed, although CCCA primarily afflicts Black Americans, one case was reported in a white woman who repeatedly used curling irons over several years [80]. Further, one study of Nigerian women found that prolonged use of chemical relaxers may be associated with the development of scarring alopecias including CCCA [112]. The etiology of CCCA is thus complex with multiple predisposing factors, and the pathogenesis is not yet entirely delineated [95].

As with other scarring alopecias, CCCA is characterized by inflammation of the hair follicle and the replacement of follicular epithelium with connective tissue [95]. Uniquely, it presents first on the vertex of the scalp and then progresses peripherally in a circular distribution over the crown [101]. Throughout the region of scarring, hair growth is sparse, short, and brittle [95]. Tenderness and pruritus may develop in the affected area as well [101]. In late stages of CCCA, scarring and hair loss become irreversible.

Scarring alopecia is permanent, so preventing further hair loss is an important goal of therapy. Physicians should recommend immediate haircare modifications including stopping use of chemical relaxers and traction-inducing hairstyles [95].

If chemical relaxers cannot be discontinued, it is suggested that patients use professional services, mild relaxers, and less frequent touch-ups to minimize the potentially damaging effect of relaxers [101]. Other habit changes include reducing use of heat and washing the hair every 1 to 2 weeks to treat any underlying seborrheic dermatitis and reduce itching and scaling.

Aggressive use of anti-inflammatory medications is another important component of treatment. Daily high-potency topical steroids and monthly intralesional corticosteroids are first line treatments [95]. Application should be targeted to the periphery of the affected area to prevent further spread. After stabilization of disease, use of topicals can be reduced to every other day; intralesional corticosteroids can be used symptomatically. Highly aggressive cases may be treated with oral agents such as tetracyclines. Responses typically occur within 6 months. After 1 year of remission, steroids may be discontinued.

Summary

Hair oils are used to soften and shine the hair as well as promote hair growth and prevent alopecia. Commonly used by Asian Indians and Black Americans, they are primarily made of hydrophobic compounds that are especially useful in fortifying ethnic hair. Oils have demonstrated anti-microbial properties as well. However, many oils can trigger allergic contact dermatitis, and organic oils may worsen seborrheic dermatitis. Mudichood can also result from use of hair oils in hot, humid climates.

Several options are available for relaxing hair, and each has its own complications. Hot comb use may lead to burns, hair breakage, and central centrifugal cicatricial alopecia. Chemical relaxers have potential side effects of seborrhea, alopecia, and irritant contact dermatitis Brazilian keratin treatments frequently contain high concentrations of formaldehyde or formaldehyde-releasing compounds. Reported complications include allergic contact dermatitis and psoriasiform eruptions.

Hairstyles worn by ethnic populations, such as tight cornrows, may also lead to development of dermatitis and alopecia. Complications of braids include traction folliculitis and alopecia, scalp cutaneous necrosis, and CCCA. Hair extensions, or weaves, may result in traction folliculitis and alopecia, CCCA, and latex allergy to the bonding glue.

References

1. Dias MFRG. Hair cosmetics: an overview. Int J Trichology. 2015;7:2–15.
2. Vashi N, et al. Dermatoses caused by cultural practices: cosmetic cultural practices. J Am Acad Dermatol. 2018;79:19–30.
3. McMichael A. Ethnic hair update: past and present. J Am Acad Dermatol. 2003;48:S127–33.
4. van der Donk J, et al. Quality of life and maladjustment associated with hair loss in. Soc Sci Med. 1994;38:159–63.
5. Williamson D, Gonzalez M, Finlay A. The effect of hair loss on quality of life. J Eur Acad Dermatol Venereol. 2000;15:137–9.
6. Morrison A. Straightening up: black women law professors, interracial relationships, and academic fit(ting) in. Harvard J Law Gender. 2010;33:85–98.
7. Greensword SN-K. Producing "fabulous": commodification and ethnicity in hair braiding salons. Baton Rouge: LSU Doctoral Dissertations; 2017.
8. Gupta D, Thappa D. Dermatoses due to Indian cultural practices. Indian J Dermatol. 2015;60:3–12.
9. Uwakwe L, McMichael A. Commonly used natural oils in hair grooming. The Dermatologist. 2018;26(5). Published online. https://www.the-dermatologist.com/issue-content/commonly-used-natural-oils-hair-grooming.
10. Orchard A, et al. The influence of carrier oils on the antimicrobial activity and cytotoxicity of essential oils. Evid Based Complement Alternat Med. 2019;2019:6981305. https://doi.org/10.1155/2019/6981305.
11. Lin T-K, Zhong L, Santiago JL. Anti-inflammatory and skin barrier repair effects of topical application of some plant oils. Int J Mol Sci. 2018;19:70.

12. Manion C, Widder R. Essentials of essential oils. Am J Health Syst Pharm. 2017;74:e153–62.

13. Orchard A, van Vuuren S. Carrier oils in dermatology. Arch Dermatol Res. 2019;311:653–72.

14. Ahmad Z. The uses and properties of almond oil. Complement Ther Clin Pract. 2010;16:10–2.

15. Guillet G, Guillet M. Percutaneous sensitization to almond oil in infancy and study of ointments in 27 children with food allergy. Allerg Immunol (Paris). 2000;32:309–11.

16. Garg A, Muller J. Inhibition of growth of dermatophytes by Indian hair oils. Mycoses. 1992;35:363–9.

17. Sarkar R, et al. Use of vegetable oils in dermatology: an overview. Int J Dermatol. 2017;56:1080–6.

18. Veraldi S, et al. Allergic contact dermatitis caused by argan oil. Dermatitis. 2016;27:391.

19. Foti C, et al. Allergic contact dermatitis caused by argan oil. Contact Dermatitis. 2014;71:183–4.

20. Astier C, et al. Anaphylaxis to argan oil. Allergy. 2010;65:662–3.

21. Panel CIRE. Final report on the safety assessment of ricinus communis (castor) seed oil, hydrogenated castor oil, glyceryl ricinoleate, glyceryl ricinoleate SE, ricinoleic acid, potassium ricinoleate, sodium ricinoleate, zinc ricinoleate, cetyl ricinoleate, ethyl ric. Int J Toxicol. 2007;26:S31–77.

22. Sowa J, Suzuki K, Tsuruta K, Akamatsu H, Matsunaga K. Allergic contact dermatitis from propylene glycol ricinoleate in a lipstick. Contact Dermatitis 2003;48:228–9.

23. Andersen KE, Nielsen R. Lipstick dermatitis related to castor oil. Contact Dermatitis. 1984;11(4):253–4.

24. Brandle I, Boujnah-Khouadja A, Foussereau J. Allergy to castor oil. Contact Dermatitis 1983;9:424–5

25. Taghipour K, Tatnall F, Orton D. Allergic axillary dermatitis due to hydrogenated castor oil in a deodorant. Contact Dermatitis 2008;58:168–9

26. Maduri V, Vedachalam A, Kiruthika S. "Castor Oil" – the culprit of acute hair felting. Int J Trichology. 2017;9:116–8.

27. Rele A, Mohile R. Effect of mineral oil, sunflower oil, and coconut oil on prevention of hair damage. J Cosmet Sci. 2003;54:175–92.

28. Verallo-Rowell V, Dillague K, Syah-Tjundawan B. Novel antibacterial and emollient effects of coconut and virgin olive oils in adult atopic dermatitis. Dermatitis. 2008;19:308–15.

29. Bergsson G, et al. Killing of Gram-positive cocci by fatty acids and monoglycerides. APMIS. 2001;109:670–8.
30. Burnett C, et al. Safety assessment of plant-derived fatty acid oils. Int J Toxicol. 2017;36:51S–129S.
31. Jacob S, Amini S. Cocamidopropyl betaine. Dermatitis. 2008;19:157–60.
32. Ananthapadmanabha K, et al. Cleansing without compromise: the impact of cleansers on the skin barrier and the technology of mild cleansing. Dermatol Ther. 2004;17(Suppl 1):16–25.
33. Foti C, et al. The role of 3-dimethylaminopropylamine and amidoamine in contact allergy to cocamidopropylbetaine. Contact Dermatitis. 2003;48:194–8.
34. Pilania R, et al. Revisiting a case of persistent pneumonia: complication of hair oil aspiration. J Pediatr Child Health. 2018;54:1284–5.
35. Habashy R, et al. Anti-inflammatory effects of jojoba liquid wax in experimental models. Pharmacol Res. 2005;51:95–105.
36. Ranzato E, Martinotti S, Burlando B. Wound healing properties of jojoba liquid wax: an in vitro study. J Ethnopharmacol. 2011;134:443–9.
37. Scott M, Scott M Jr. Jojoba oil. J Am Acad Dermatol. 1982;6:545.
38. Di Berardino L, et al. A case of contact dermatitis from jojoba. Contact Dermatitis. 2006;55:57–8.
39. Wantke F, et al. Contact dermatitis from jojoba oil and myristyllactate/maleated soybean oil. Contact Dermatitis. 1996;34:71–2.
40. Pasricha J, Gupta R, Gupta S. Contact hypersensitaity to mustard khal and mustard oil. Indian J Dermatol Venereol Leprol. 1985;51:108–10.
41. Zawar V. Pityriasis rosea-like eruptions due to mustard oil application. Indian J Dermatol Venereol Leprol. 2005;71:282–4.
42. Siegfried E, Glenn E. Use of olive oil for the treatment of seborrheic dermatitis in children. Arch Pediatr Adolesc Med. 2012;166:967.
43. Dawson T Jr. Malassezia globosa and restricta: breakthrough understanding of the etiology and treatment of dandruff and seborrheic dermatitis through whole-genome analysis. J Investig Dermatol Symp Proc. 2007;12:15–9.
44. de Groot A, Schmidt E. Essential oils, part V: peppermint oil, lavender oil, and lemongrass oil. Dermatitis. 2016;27:325–32.
45. Wu P, James W. Lavender. Dermatitis. 2011;22:344–7.

46. Schaller M, Korting H. Allergic airborne contact dermatitis from essential oils used in aromatherapy. Clin Exp Dermatol. 1995;20:143–5.

47. Varma S, et al. Combined contact allergy to tea tree oil and lavender oil complicating chronic vulvovaginitis. Contact Dermatitis. 2000;42:309–10.

48. Goiriz R, et al. Photoallergic contact dermatitis from lavender oil in topical ketoprofen. Contact Dermatitis. 2007;57:381–2.

49. Matthieu L, et al. Contact and photocontact allergy to ketoprofen. The Belgian experience. Contact Dermatitis. 2004;50:238–41.

50. Brandao F. Occupational allergy to lavender oil. Contact Dermatitis. 1986;15:249–50.

51. Bleasel N, Tate B, Rademaker M. Allergic contact dermatitis following exposure to essential oils. Australas J Dermatol. 2002;43:211–3.

52. Boonchai W, Iamtharachai P, Sunthonpalin P. Occupational allergic contact dermatitis from essential oils in aromatherapists. Contact Dermatitis. 2007;56:181–2.

53. Tratter A, David M, Lazarov A. Occupational contact dermatitis due to essential oils. Contact Dermatitis. 2008;58:282–4.

54. Skold M, et al. Studies on the autoxidation and sensitizing capacity of the fragrance chemical linalool, identifying a linalool hydroperoxide. Contact Dermatitis. 2002;46:267–72.

55. Skol M, Hagvall L, Karlberg A. Autoxidation of linalyl acetate, the main component of lavender oil, creates potent contact allergens. Contact Dermatitis. 2008;58:9–14.

56. Hagvall L, et al. Lavender oil lacks natural protection against autoxidation, forming strong contact allergens on air exposure. Contact Dermatitis. 2008;59:143–50.

57. de Groot A, Schmidt E. Tea tree oil: contact allergy and chemical composition. Contact Dermatitis. 2016;75:129–43.

58. Homer L, et al. Natural variation in the essential oil content of Melaleuca alternifolia Cheel (Myrtaceae). Biochem Syst Ecol. 2000;28:367–82.

59. Satchell A, et al. Treatment of dandruff with 5% tea tree oil shampoo. J Am Acad Dermatol. 2002;47:852–5.

60. Buck D, Nidorf D, Addino J. Comparison of two topical preparations for the treatment of onychomycosis: Melaleuca alternifolia (tea tree) oil and clotrimazole. J Fam Pract. 1994;38:601–5.

61. Carson C, Hammer K, Riley T. Melaleuca alternifolia (Tea Tree) oil: a review of antimicrobial and other medicinal properties. Clin Microbiol Rev. 2006;19:50–62.
62. Hammer K, Carson C, Riley T. Antifungal effects of Melaleuca alternifolia (tea tree) oil and its components on Candida albicans, Candida glabrata and Saccharomyces cerevisiae. J Antimicrob Chemother. 2004;53:1081–5.
63. Cox S, et al. The mode of antimicrobial action of the essential oil of Melaleuca alternifolia (tea tree oil). J Appl Microbiol. 2000;88:170–5.
64. Carson C, et al. Susceptibility of methicillin-resistant Staphylococcus aureus to the essential oil of Melaleuca alternifolia. J Antimicrob Chemother. 1995;35:421–4.
65. Schnitzler P, Schon K, Reichling J. Antiviral activity of Australian tea tree oil and eucalyptus oil against herpes simplex virus in cell culture. Pharmazie. 2001;56:343–7.
66. Mikus J, et al. In vitro effect of essential oils and isolated mono- and sesquiterpenes on Leishmania major and Trypanosoma brucei. Planta Med. 2000;66:366–8.
67. Koh K, et al. Tea tree oil reduces histamine-induced skin inflammation. Br J Dermatol. 2002;147:1212–7.
68. Khalil Z, et al. Regulation of wheal and flare by tea tree oil: complementary human and rodent studies. J Investig Dermatol. 2004;123:683–90.
69. Hausen B. Kontaktallergie auf Teebaumöl und Ascaridol. Akt Dermatol. 1998;24:60–2.
70. Harkenthal M, Hausen G, Reichling J. 1,2,4-Trihydroxy menthane, a contact allergen from oxidized Australian tea tree oil. Pharmazie. 2000;55:153–4.
71. Roy R, Thakur M, Dixit V. Development and evaluation of polyherbal formulation for hair growth-promoting activity. J Cosmet Dermatol. 2007;6:108–12.
72. Jahan R, et al. Ethnopharmacological significance of Eclipta alba (L.) Hassk. (Asteraceae). Int Sch Res Notices. 2014;2014:385969. https://doi.org/10.1155/2014/385969. eCollection 2014.
73. Sugathan P. Mudi-chood disease. Dermatol Online J. 1999;5:5.
74. Kumar D, et al. Novel dermoscopic findings in mudi-chood disease – a case report. Int J Dermatol. 2017;56:776–8.
75. Ashique K. Mudi-chood: an interesting dermatological entity. Int J Dermatol. 2015;54:806.

76. Gupta G, et al. Mudichood: well-known but rare entity. Int J Trichology. 2013;5:101.
77. Vashi NA. Dermatoanthropology of ethnic skin and hair. Boston: Springer International Publishing; 2017.
78. Etemesi BA. Impact of hair relaxers in women in Nakuru, Kenya. Int J Dermatol. 2007;46(Suppl 1):23–5.
79. Syed A. Ethnic hair care: history, trends and formulation. Cosmet Toil. 1993;108:99–107.
80. LoPresti P, Papa C, Kligman A. Hot comb alopecia. Arch Dermatol. 1968;98:234–8.
81. de Sá Dias T, et al. Relaxing/straightening of Afro-ethnic hair: historical overview. J Cosmet Dermatol. 2007;6:2–5.
82. Shetty V, Shetty N, Nair D. Chemical hair relaxers have adverse effects a myth or reality. Int J Dermatol. 2013;5:26–8.
83. Khumalo N, Pillay K, Ngwanya R. Acute 'relaxer'-associated scarring alopecia: a report of five cases. Br J Dermatol. 2007;156:1394–7.
84. Kaur B, Singh H, Lin-Greenberg A. Irritant contact dermatitis complicated by deep-seated staphylococcal infection caused by a hair relaxer. J Natl Med Assoc. 2002;94:121–3.
85. Wise L, et al. Hair relaxer use and risk of uterine leiomyomata in African-American women. Am J Epidemiol. 2012;175:432–40.
86. Booker M. Stevens-Johnson syndrome triggered by chemical hair relaxer: a case report. Cases J. 2009;2:7748.
87. Weathersby C, McMichael A. Brazilian keratin hair treatment: an review. J Cosmet Dermatol. 2013;12:144–8.
88. Manelli M, Smith P, Khumalo N. Elevated formaldehyde concentration in "Brazilian keratin type" hair-straightening products: a cross-sectional study. J Am Acad Dermatol. 2014;70:276–80.
89. Simpson W, Crawshaw G. Wool: science and technology. Boca Raton: Woodhead Publishing Ltd.; 2002.
90. United States Department of Labor, O.a.S.H.A. Hair salons: facts about formaldehyde in hair smoothing products. Washington, DC: United States Department of Labor, Occupational and Safety Health Administration; 2012.
91. Pierce J, et al. Characterization of formaldehyde exposure resulting from the use of four professional hair straightening products. J Occup Environ Hyg. 2011;8:686–99.
92. Gavazzoni-Dias M, et al. Eczema-like psoriasiform skin reaction due to Brazilian keratin treatment. Skin Appendage Disord. 2016;1:156–62.

93. Van Lerberghe L, Baeck M. A case of acute contact dermatitis induced by formaldehyde in hair-straightening products. Contact Dermatitis. 2014;70:384–6.
94. Kyei A, Bergfeld WF, Piliang M. Medical and environmental risk factors for the development of central centrifugal cicatricial alopecia. Arch Dermatol. 2011;147(8):909–14.
95. Gathers RC, Lim H. Central centrifugal cicatricial alopecia: past, present, and future. J Am Acad Dermatol. 2009;60:660–8.
96. Salibi A, Soueid A, Dancey A. Hair braiding (plaiting) and hair extensions: an underestimated danger! J Plast Reconstr Aesthet Surg. 2014;67:e206–7.
97. Borab Z, et al. Hair braiding-induced scalp necrosis: a case report. Eplasty. 2016;16:ic14.
98. Raffini L, Tsarouhas N. Subgaleal hematoma from hair braiding leads to the diagnosis of von Willebrand disease. Pediatr Emerg Care. 2004;20:316–8.
99. Vu T, et al. Subgaleal hematoma from hair braiding: case report and literature review. Pediatr Emerg Care. 2004;20:821–3.
100. Adeloya A, Odeku E. Subgaleal hematoma in head injuries. Int Surg. 1975;60:263–5.
101. Callender V, McMichael A, Cohen G. Medical and surgical therapies for alopecias in black women. Dermatol Ther. 2004;17(2):164–76.
102. Grimes P, Davis L. Cosmetics in blacks. Dermatol Clin. 1991;9:53–68.
103. Cogen F, Beezhold D. Hair glue anaphylaxis: a hidden latex allergy. Ann Allergy Asthma Immunol. 2002;88:61–3.
104. Rudolph R, Klein A, Decherd JW. Corn-row alopecia. Arch Dermatol. 1973;108:134.
105. Halder R. Hair and scalp disorders in blacks. Cutis. 1983;32:378–80.
106. Kanwar A, et al. Traction alopecia in Sikh males. Arch Dermatol. 1989;125:1587.
107. Singh G. Letter: traction alopecia in Sikh boys. Br J Dermatol. 1975;92:232–3.
108. Samrao A, et al. The "Fringe Sign" – a useful clinical finding in traction alopecia of the marginal hair line. Dermatol Online J. 2011;17:1.
109. McMichael A. Hair and scalp disorders in ethnic populations. Dermatol Clin. 2003;21:629–44.

110. Earles R. Surgical correction of traumatic alopecia marginalis or traction alopecia in black women. J Dermatol Surg Oncol. 1986;12:78–82.
111. Sperling L, Cowper S. The histopathology of primary cicatricial alopecia. Semin Cutan Med Surg. 2006;25:41–50.
112. Nnoruka N. Hair loss: is there a relationship with hair care practices in Nigeria? Int J Dermatol. 2005;44:13–7.

Chapter 4
Religious Dermatoses

Nicole Trepanowski, Nicole Patzelt, and Neelam A. Vashi

Dermatologic complications can arise due to the events that take place in the practice of various religions. As the world is becoming more culturally diverse, it is important for dermatologists to be aware of religious dermatoses and how they might present. A knowledge and understanding of basic religious practices will help dermatologists better serve the needs of their patients as well as provide proper counseling and management to help treat these conditions. Without

N. Trepanowski
Boston University School of Medicine, Boston, MA, USA

N. Patzelt
Department of Dermatology, Boston Medical Center, Boston, MA, USA

N. A. Vashi (✉)
Boston University School of Medicine, Boston, MA, USA

Department of Dermatology, Boston Medical Center, Boston, MA, USA

Department of Dermatology, Boston University Center for Ethnic Skin, Boston, MA, USA

Boston University Cosmetic and Laser Center, Boston, MA, USA

Department of Veteran Affairs, Boston Health Care System, Boston, MA, USA

© The Author(s) 2021
N. A. Vashi (ed.), *Cultural Practices and Dermatoses*,
https://doi.org/10.1007/978-3-030-68992-6_4

79

exposure or background, dermatologists are unlikely to ask about the religious practices of their patients, and will thus lack important diagnostic information essential for the care and treatment of their patients.

In this chapter, we discuss several religious practices with dermatologic complications. We will be discussing the dermatoses associated with the following religions: Hinduism, Buddhism, Islam, Sikhism, Judaism, and Christianity. It is important to recognize that sometimes cultural and religious practices are intertwined. For example, we will discuss the use of betel quid in Buddhism that is also used for social purposes (breath refreshment). Thus, the following dermatoses may not be limited to only those that practice the religion that they are associated with.

The following conditions draw from published case reports and series on religious dermatologic complications. A lack of published data and formal studies on religious dermatoses limit conclusions regarding prevalence of these conditions.

This chapter is divided into different subsections based on the religion associated with each dermatologic condition. Information on the background, complications, and treatment of each religious dermatosis is provided. Table 4.1 includes a summary of various religious dermatoses, their associated religion(s), prevention, and treatment options.

Hinduism

Alta Dermatitis

Background

Hindu women use alta, a red dye, to color their feet during religious celebrations. Preparations of alta have been found to contain the azo dyes Crocein Scarlet MOO and Solvent Yellow 3, which form breakdown products that are toxic to melanocytes when exposed to the environment [1, 2].

TABLE 4.1 Summary of religious dermatoses

Religion of origin	Form of worship/ celebration	Mechanism/Definition	Dermatologic complications	Prevention	Treatment
Hinduism	Alta	Red dye applied to the feet during religious festivals, consisting of dyes that form melanocytotoxic metabolites [1, 2]	Allergic and irritant contact dermatitis and chemical leukoderma [2, 3]	Avoidance of exposure or switching to a chemical-free formulation	Depigmentation is rarely reversible [2]
Hinduism	Holi	Spring festival, participants throw colors on each other consisting of artificial dyes [4, 5]	Allergic contact dermatitis, urticaria, secondary pyoderma, xerosis, periorbital necrotizing fasciitis, conjunctival discoloration, temporary vision loss [4–8]	Avoidance of exposure	Short dose of topical corticosteroids [4, 6]

(continued)

TABLE 4.1 (continued)

Religion of origin	Form of worship/ celebration	Mechanism/Definition	Dermatologic complications	Prevention	Treatment
Hinduism, Islam	Kalava	Ritual thread tied tightly around the wrist during religious and cultural celebrations [9, 10]	Inflammation, foreign body granuloma, scar [9]	Tie the thread less tightly	Remove foreign body material, topical antibiotic, topical corticosteroids. Systemic corticosteroids if warranted [9]
Hinduism, Buddhism	Betel quid	Betel leaves, areca nut mixture chewed during religious ceremonies. Arecoline, arecaidine, elevated copper levels, fibroblast activation, fibrinogen degradation products, and excessive fibrin deposition may contribute to pathogenesis [11–16]	Oral submucous fibrosis, periodontal disease, dental caries, leukoplakia, lichenoid lesions, hyper and hyposalivation, oral squamous cell carcinoma, pharyngeal and esophageal carcinoma [14, 18–23]	Avoidance of exposure, educate patient on risks of use.	Antifibrotic compounds such as tanshinone IIA/salvianolic acid A/salvianolic acid B may treat oral submucous fibrosis but not yet tested in humans [13]

Islam, Buddhism	Prayer marks	Five daily prayers in various positions lasting 5–10 minutes each causing repetitive friction and pressure [24, 25]	Thickening, hyperpigmentation, lichenification, callus, and/or frictional melanosis on bridge of the nose, forehead, knees, ankles, and dorsa of the feet [24, 26, 27]	Incorporate soft prayer rugs and thick clothing over bony prominences, modify stances if possible [28]	May spontaneously regress, removal of nodules using surgical curettage after softening with 40% urea or topical keratolytics [28, 29]
Islam	Headscarves	Religious attire wrapped around the head and upper torso and secured with plastic or metal safety pins [32]	Vitiligo, depigmentation, and/ or lichen simplex chronicus [32]	Change method and location of securing the scarf [32].	Change method and location of securing the scarf [32]

(continued)

TABLE 4.1 (continued)

Religion of origin	Form of worship/ celebration	Mechanism/Definition	Dermatologic complications	Prevention	Treatment
Islam	Orf	Sacrifice of infected sheep or goats for the Feast of Sacrifice results in animal-human transmission of Orf [33–35]	Phlegmonous or ulceratovegative lesions, and/or cellulitis, generally on the hands [35]	Education on prevention of viral transmission, encourage glove usage and hand washing [35]	Often spontaneously remits, topical antibiotic, systemic antibiotic, or surgical excision if necessary [36]
Sikhism	Turban ear	Sikh men tie their long hair into a tight knot and wrap a turban around it. They also tie their beards into a tight knot. Both of these techniques cause excessive pressure on the ears [37–39]	Perichondritis, chondrodermatitis nodularis helicis, hyperpigmentation, nodules, and/or ulceration on the ears [40, 41]	Wrap the hair less tightly, wear the hair loose, and/ or remove the turban at night [37–39, 41]	Topical and intralesional steroids, topical 2% glycerol trinitrate, CO2 laser, surgical excision of the cartilage, and curettage [41]

| Sikhism | Traction alopecia | Sikh men tie their long hair into a tight knot and wrap a turban around it. They also tie their beards into a tight knot. Both of these techniques cause excessive pressure on the hair follicles [37–39] | Traction alopecia on the sides of the mandible and the frontoparietal scalp, scarring alopecia [37–39] | Wrap the hair less tightly, wear the hair loose, and/ or remove the turban at night [37–39, 41] | Restorative hair transplantation [38] |
| Judaism | Davener's dermatosis | Jewish prayer method involving repetitive swaying leading to constant friction and damage of the stratum corneum and melanocyte stimulation [42, 43] | Asymptomatic elongated, longitudinal, hyperpigmented patches overlying the inferior thoracic and superior lumbar vertebrae [42] | Avoidance of exposure, wearing thick, protective clothing over the exposed area, and covering the back of the chair with protective material | Chemical peels, lightening creams, erbium-doped fractional photothermolysis, and Q- switched lasers [43] |

(continued)

TABLE 4.1 (continued)

Religion of origin	Form of worship/ celebration	Mechanism/Definition	Dermatologic complications	Prevention	Treatment
Judaism	Phylactery dermatitis	A religious ornament that is wrapped around the forehead and secured with leather straps that fall onto the neck and anterior waist. Another ornament is wrapped around the left upper arm with leather straps that trail to the fingers. Allergens on the straps are believed to be the cause of the allergic contact dermatitis [44–48]	Allergic contact dermatitis [44–48]	Wrap the phylactery in plastic wrap to avoid skin contact with the potential allergens, avoid wearing the phylactery, or use alternate allergen-free versions when possible [47]	Mid-potency corticosteroids and antihistamines [47]

Christianity	Pew blisters	Christians kneel on pews for extended periods of time during church services and other times of worship, causing extended periods of friction [49]	Blisters, bullae, and/or calluses [50, 51]	Avoidance of kneeling, wearing thick protective clothing over exposed areas, placing a soft rug or mat on the pew to reduce pressure [50]	Avoidance of kneeling, wearing thick protective clothing over exposed areas, placing a soft rug or mat on the pew to reduce pressure [50]
Christianity	Holy week hypertrich-osis	*Costaleros* in Spain carry statues on their shoulders during the holy week and practice throughout the year, causing extended friction [52]	Hypertrichosis overlying a firm mass [53]	Cessation of weight-bearing on affected area [53]	Cessation of weight-bearing on affected area [53]

Complications

Adverse events associated with the use of alta include allergic and irritant contact dermatitis and chemical leukoderma on the sides of the feet and toes and dorsa of the feet. Patients may initially present with hyperpigmentation, pruritus, and scaling on the affected areas [3]. Continued use of alta can lead to depigmentation of affected areas [2].

Treatment

The treatment of alta dermatitis proves difficult as it is generally non-reversible [2]. Cessation of the use of alta or switching to a chemical-free or alternate formulation may help prevent further damage.

Holi Dermatoses

Background

Holi is a religious festival that occurs in the Spring where participants celebrate a year of fertility and harvest. Participants throw colored pastes, dyes, watercolors, and powders on family, friends, and strangers at large gatherings [4]. Traditionally practiced in India, Holi has now become a popular celebration on American college campuses. It is important to recognize that non-Hindus also participate in the festivities, and may present with Holi-associated dermatoses.

In the past, the dyes used for Holi were traditionally prepared from flowers and trees thought to have Ayurvedic medicinal properties. Now, commercially produced dyes are commonly used, including copper sulfate and malachite green (green), mercury sulfate (red), cobalt nitrate, Prussian blue, indigo/zinc salts (blue), aluminum bromide (silver), and zinc oxide (black) [4, 5]. To produce a glittering effect, silica, mica, and asbestos dust are often added to the preparations [4].

Complications

In the weeks following the Holi festivities, an annual increase in allergic contact dermatitis and other dermatoses has been observed in festival participants. Patients may present with pruritus, oozing, pain, burning, and scaling. Lesions on exposed areas such as the face, dorsum of the hands, palmar surface of the hands, forearms, arms, trunk, and scalp can be erythematous, urticarial, eczematous, and xerotic. The nail folds may become acutely inflamed, and secondary infections may also occur. In areas where liquid dyes pool, severe lesions can develop. Preexisting dermatologic conditions such as acne, chronic paronychia, and eczema may become acutely exacerbated [4, 5]. Ocular complications include conjunctival discoloration, erythema, pain, watering, itching, temporary vision loss, periorbital necrotizing fasciitis, and grittiness [5–8].

Treatment

These conditions, termed "Holi dermatoses", typically respond well to a short dose of topical corticosteroid [4, 6].

Kalava Induced Foreign Body Granuloma

Background

Kalava, also known as kalawa or kautuka, is a sacred ritual thread tied around the wrist during Hindu and Muslim religious and cultural celebrations [9, 10]. Men, women, and children wear the kalava for different ceremonies.

Complications

Tightly tied kalava has caused complications in children. Because of religious beliefs, parents may not immediately untie the thread. In these circumstances, inflammation and pain develop on the affected area in the following weeks. On occasion, the threads of kalava have penetrated the injury site leading to the formation of foreign body granuloma [9]. The inflammation associated with kalava typically resolves within 2 weeks, but severe cases can lead to scar formation [9].

Treatment

Treatment includes removal of any foreign body material, a topical antibiotic, and a topical corticosteroid. Systemic corticosteroids may be given if warranted [9].

Buddhism

Betel Quid

Background

Betel quid is a combination of betel leaves and areca nuts originally employed as a religious offering in Hindu and Buddhist ceremonies. Betel quid now often contains fillers/ flavorings including tobacco and other spices. The use of betel quid is no longer constrained to religious offerings as now people of various religious backgrounds use betel quid because of its stimulant, breath-refreshing, and anti-helminthic properties [11, 12].

Complications

Chewing betel quid can lead to oral submucosal fibrosis, a chronic and precancerous lesion of the oral mucosa. The pathogenesis of oral submucosal fibrosis attributed to betel quid is thought to be due to the release of the compounds arecoline and arecaidine [13]. In addition, elevated copper levels, fibroblast activation, fibrinogen degradation products, and excessive fibrin deposition may also contribute to its pathogenesis [14–16]. Patients may present with difficulty opening their mouth and describe a burning sensation. The oral mucosa may be covered with white, fibrous bands [13]. The risk of oral submucosal fibrosis increases with frequency of use as well as duration [17]. Discoloration of dental and oral mucosa, oral leukoplakia, periodontal disease, dental caries, lichenoid lesions, and hyper- and hyposalivation are other complications associated with the use of betel quid [18–21]. One study found that 11.7% of betel quid users had oral leukoplakia and 6.1% had oral submucous fibrosis [18]. The prolonged chemical and mechanical irritation associated with the use of betel quid may transform this condition into oral squamous cell cancer at a rate of 3–19% [14]. Other cancers associated with the use of betel quid include pharyngeal and esophageal cancers. The concurrent use of tobacco products and alcohol consumption raises an individual's risk for these cancers [22, 23].

Treatment

Antifibrotic compounds such as tanshinone IIA/salvianolic acid A/salvianolic acid B may treat oral submucous fibrosis but not yet tested in humans [13]. Educating the patient on the risks of chewing betel quid is imperative to prevent the development of cancer attributed to betel quid.

Islam

Prayer Marks

Background

The second pillar of Islam is called Salat. Salat consists of a series of prayer positions called Waquf (standing), Ruku (bowing), Sajda (prostration), and Julus (sitting), each lasting between 5 and 10 minutes [24]. Salat is a ritual that should be performed five times daily by all Muslims in normal circumstances [25]. An individual may wash their hands prior to each prayer.

Complications

The prayer method utilized in the practice of Islam can lead to the development of prayer marks, also known as prayer nodules or prayer hyperpigmentation. Individuals develop asymptomatic skin changes on bony prominences such as the forehead, bridge of the nose, knees, ankles, and dorsa of the feet due to the repetitive pressure from the prayer stances. These asymptomatic skin changes can include hyperpigmentation, thickening, and lichenification [24, 26, 27]. The prayer marks are initially mobile, smooth, and soft, but can develop into a callus [24]. The forehead may develop frictional melanosis. Hand dermatitis may occur due to the frequent hand-washing that occurs with each set of prayers.

Prayer marks are most commonly found on the knees and feet bilaterally. The left foot is often frequently involved due to the posture during the Julus (sitting) stance. The incidence of prayer marks increases with age; the lowest incidence is among those 20–25 years of age, and the highest incidence is among those 50 and older. Females are less likely to develop prayer marks than men, and their prayer markers are often less severe. This is postulated to be due to the fact that females have more subcutaneous tissue protecting their bony prominences, spend less time practicing Salat, and have less sun exposure [24].

Prayer marks are not limited to the practice of Islam. They have also been reported on the lateral malleoli of a Buddhist monk who meditated cross-legged for several consecutive days [28].

The development of prayer marks in unusual locations may provide additional information regarding a patient's systemic health [29, 30]. For example, Cangiano et al. described a patient experiencing worsening shortness of breath due to his chronic obstructive pulmonary disease.

Additional questioning revealed that the patient developed prayer marks on his elbows (an unusual site for prayer marks) because of his need to maneuver himself in a different manner to perform his prayer rituals due to his worsening shortness of breath [30].

Treatment

In individuals who are no longer able to pray regularly, prayer marks have regressed on their own [31]. Nodules may be treated surgically, with topicals such as 40% urea, curettage, or other keratolytics [28]. Patients may modify their positioning during prayer stances, wear thick clothing covering their bony prominences, or incorporate a prayer rug into their practice [28].

Headscarf Use

Background

Headscarves are a common religious garment worn by Muslim women that cover the head, scalp, and upper torso. Metal or plastic safety pins are often used to secure the scarf in place over the center of the neck, specifically in the area of the thyroid cartilage [32].

Complications

Some Muslim women have presented with vitiligo and depigmentation over the region where they had been securing their headscarves with safety pins [32]. This melanocyte loss has been attributed to chronic pressure, minor mechanical trauma, and repeated friction from the safety pins [32]. Lichen simplex chronicus has also been associated with headscarf use [32].

Treatment

The recommended treatment involves changing the method and location of securing the scarf [32].

Orf

Background

The Muslim Feast of Sacrifice, also known as Eid-al-Adha or Eid-al-Kebir, is a religious celebration that occurs annually 2 months and 10 days after the end of Ramadan. Each Muslim family kills a lamb or sheep during this feast, and the animal is bled alive as a part of the ritual [33–35]. This method results in close contact with the animal, facilitating the transmission of virus from sheep to humans [33]. Specifically, Orf, also known as ecthyma contagiosum, is a cutaneous infection caused by a poxvirus that is transmitted to humans via contact with infected sheep and goats [34].

Complications

Infections with Orf following the observance of the Muslim Feast of Sacrifice typically occur in the days to weeks following the religious observance [33]. Orf causes infection by entering through skin lesions, often caused by knife handling during the slaughter, or pre-existing skin lesions [35]. Orf most commonly causes lesions on the hands [35]. Patients may present with fever, malaise, phlegmonous lesions, ulceratovegetative lesions, and cellulitis [35]. The skin lesions associated with Orf virus infection are often polymorphous and may consist of vesicles, blisters, pustules, erosions, ulcers, papules, and nodules [36]. Patients may present with a single lesion or multiple lesions [35]. Only men are traditionally allowed to sacrifice the sheep, but infections have been noted in women or children who had contact with the skin and meat of the animal [33, 35]. Infection can be detected using PCR, viral culture, or EM [35].

Treatment

Orf spontaneously remits within 6 weeks, but lingering pain, bacterial superinfections, and regional lymphadenitis are possible complications [36]. Treatment includes the application of topical antiseptics and prophylactic systemic antibiotics if deemed necessary [36]. Treatment of Orf may also require surgical excision [35]. It is important to educate patients on the potential for virus transmission and methods to avoid infection [35]. Patients that will handle animals for the Feast of Sacrifice should be encouraged to wear gloves, avoid exposure to open skin wounds, and wash hands thoroughly with soap and water after contacting animals [35].

Sikhism

Turban Ear

Background

A turban is a form of head attire that consists of a long piece of cloth tightly wrapped around the head. The original holy gurus of Sikhism were given a turban to disguise their uncut hair. Men and women who practice Sikhism follow this tradition and do not cut their hair as a symbol of religious devotion. Men tie their hair into a tight knot on the frontal scalp with a handkerchief or 'guti' placed on top of the knot before covering the hair with a turban for lengthy periods of time [37, 38]. Men also tie their beard hair into a tight knot [37, 39].

Complications

Turban use can lead to the development of turban ear, which consists of lesions on the ears ranging from perichondritis to chondrodermatitis nodularis helicis attributed to prolonged pressure and trauma [40, 41]. Patients may present with a range of symptoms varying from non-bothersome tenderness to intense pain exacerbated when sleeping [40, 41]. Hyperpigmentation, notable skin markings, firm erythematous nodules, and ultimately ulceration have been noted on the bilateral tragi and antihelices [40, 41].

Treatment

Treatment of turban ear includes reducing the pressure on the ears caused by the turban [37–39, 41]. A physician can recommend that the patient wrap the hair less tightly, wear the hair loose, or remove the turban at night. Topical and intralesional steroids, topical 2% glycerol trinitrate, CO_2 laser, surgical excision of the cartilage, and curettage may be employed to treat the secondary skin changes associated with turban use [41].

Traction Alopecia from Turban Use

Background

As discussed in the previous section, male Sikhs wear turbans tightly wrapped around their heads and refrain from cutting their hair as a form of religious devotion.

Complications

The tightly wrapped hair beneath Sikh turbans and tightly wound beard hair causes prolonged mechanical stress on the hair follicles, leading to traction alopecia in some instances. The location of the traction alopecia is generally along the sides of the mandible and the frontoparietal scalp [37–39]. Traction alopecia is considered reversible, but it may result in scarring if left untreated.

Treatment

Treatment for traction alopecia involves reducing the physical stress on the hair follicles [37–39, 41]. Similar to the treatment for turban ear, patients should be encouraged to tie their hair less tightly and wear their hair turban-free whenever possible. If the condition progresses to scarring alopecia, the only definitive treatment is restorative hair transplantation [38].

Judaism

Davener's Dermatosis

Background

Davening is a Jewish prayer method where young male Jewish students discuss, recite texts, and pray from the Torah in Orthodox Jewish Talmudic seminaries, also known as Yeshivas. These students spend hours swaying their upper chests back and forth in a rhythmic motion against a rigid backboard, symbolizing a flickering candle flame. The students are generally seated in hard chairs made of wood or metal [42].

Complications

Davener's dermatosis is a frictional melanosis [42]. The prolonged friction during lengthy prayer sessions is thought to stimulate melanocyte division while damaging the stratum corneum, reducing function of deeper keratinocytes and melanocytes. Melanin is thus lost into the papillary dermis [43].

Patients are generally asymptomatic and unaware of their lesions which may be discovered on routine skin exam overlying the spinal processes of the inferior thoracic and superior lumbar vertebrae [42]. The lesions consist of elongated, longitudinal, hyperpigmented patches. Lesions may be mild and consist of a cobblestoned appearance of 'islands' of minimal hyperpigmentation with inconclusive borders. Severe lesions can take a continuous appearance with heavier pigmentation, well-defined borders, and mild induration [42].

Treatment

Treatment includes avoiding the physical stressor, wearing thick protective clothing over the affected area when participating in Davening, or covering the back of the chair with material to reduce the friction. To treat the hyperpigmentation, chemical peels, lightening creams, erbium-doped fractional photothermolysis, and Q-switched lasers may be employed [43].

Phylactery Dermatitis

Background

A phylactery, also termed tefillin, is a religious ornament donned by Jewish men during their non-holiday, weekday, morning prayers. A phylactery has two components. A box containing parchment with biblical script is wrapped around the forehead and secured with leather straps around the head that fall onto the neck and anterior waist. Another box is wrapped around the left upper arm with leather straps that trail down the arms to the fingers [44, 45].

Complications

Wearing a phylactery has been associated with the development of allergic contact dermatitis. Patients may present with erythematous, pruritic eruptions in a spiral pattern on the posterior neck and down the left arm [44]. Ethyl acrylate 0.1%, potassium dichromate, methyl methyl-methacrylate 2%, formaldehyde, *p*-tertiary butylphenol formaldehyde resin 1%, colophonium, and *p*-phenylenediamine 1% are allergens that have been implicated [44–48].

Treatment

Patients should be encouraged to wrap their phylactery in plastic wrap to avoid skin contact with the potential allergens, avoid wearing the phylactery, or use alternate allergen-free versions. Treatment of the allergic contact dermatitis may include mid-potency corticosteroids and antihistamines [47].

Christianity

Pew Blisters

Background

Christians kneel on pews during church services as an expression of worship, humility, and submission [49]. Christians may attend church services weekly or more frequently if attending a parochial school or for other devotional purposes. Church services tend to last between 1 and 2 hours, with the amount of time spent kneeling differing on the specific service as well as the particular sect of Christianity.

Complications

Pew blisters, also referred to as prayer blisters, is a frictional dermatoses seen among Christians. Bullae and/or calluses may develop on the bilateral knees after repetitive and frequent kneeling during church services. In particular, pew blisters have been associated with the Roman Catholic sect of Christianity [50, 51].

Treatment

Similar to other frictional dermatoses mentioned in this chapter, a physician may recommend stopping or reducing the repetitive motion of kneeling, wearing special protective clothing on exposed areas, or placing a soft rug or mat on the pew to reduce friction [50].

Holy Week Hypertrichosis

Background

Semana Santa, or Holy Week, is a weeklong celebration that occurs in Spain annually from Palm Sunday to Easter Sunday. Throughout the week, *costaleros* carry large statues (*pasos*) through the streets of Spain in a series of processions to celebrate the passion of Christ. The long beam of the *pasos* is carried on the shoulders of the *costaleros* for many hours. There are between 20 and 40 *costaleros* per float. The *costaleros* practice throughout the year to ensure a smooth procession. They practice with the *paso* itself as well as lift weights to prepare their bodies [52].

Complications

Holy week hypertrichosis is a friction dermatosis consisting of hypertrichosis on the inferior, posterior neck of the *costaleros* who carry *pasos* during Semana Santa [53]. Patients may have a 'costal', which is a hard, oval, mobile, subcutaneous mass with coarse, long hair emerging from the mass [53]. It is believed that the repeated year-long repetitive friction results in inflammation and hair growth [53].

Treatment

Treatment may involve recommendation of cessation of weight bearing exercises on the affected region [53].

Conclusion

In this chapter we discuss various dermatoses associated with the practice of different religions. As the world is becoming a more diverse place, it is important for physicians to be aware of the various cultural practices of their patients to provide them with the best treatment. Many of these religious dermatoses are only diagnosed when taking a thorough patient history, as their presentation can be similar to general dermatoses. Therefore, it is important for physicians to inquire about daily repetitive practices, holiday celebrations, and recent exposures.

Patients may be unaware that their religious practice is causing their dermatologic lesion, or they are aware and seeking reassurance, or the patient is aware and unbothered by their lesion. As some of these dermatoses are caused by important practices critical to their religion, patients may be unwilling to change their inciting behavior. It is important for the physician to work with the patient to discover the best individual treatment plan for that patient. Depending on patient willingness to change, different clothes, prayer rugs, dyes, hair/scarf tying techniques, among others, are to be encouraged.

References

1. Bajaj AK, Saraswat A, Srivastav PK. Chemical leucoderma: Indian scenario, prognosis, and treatment. Indian J Dermatol. 2010;55:250–4.
2. Ghosh SK, Bandyopadhyay D. Chemical leukoderma induced by colored strings. J Am Acad Dermatol. 2009;61:909–10.
3. Bajaj AK, Pandey RK, Misra K, Chatterji AK, Tiwari A, Basu S. Contact depigmentation caused by an azo dye in alta. Contact Dermatitis. 1998;38:189–93.
4. Ghosh SK, Bandyopadhyay D, Chatterjee G, Saha D. The 'holi' dermatoses: annual spate of skin diseases following the spring festival in India. Indian J Dermatol. 2009;54:240–2.

5. Ghosh SK, Bandyopadhyay D, Verma SB. Cultural practice and dermatology: the "Holi" dermatoses. Int J Dermatol. 2012;51:1385–7.

6. Gupta D, Thappa DM. Dermatoses due to Indian cultural practices. Indian J Dermatol. 2015;60:3–12.

7. Chauhan D, Arora R, Das S, Shroff D, Narula R. Bilateral periorbital necrotizing fasciitis following exposure to Holi colors: a case report. Indian J Ophthalmol. 2007;55:373–4.

8. Velpandian T, Saha K, Ravi AK, Kumari SS, Biswas NR, Ghose S. Ocular hazards of the colors used during the festival-of-colors (Holi) in India—malachite green toxicity. J Hazard Mater. 2007;139:204–8.

9. Misri R, Jakhar D, Gupta R, Kumar S. Kalava induced foreign body reaction. J Am Acad Dermatol. 2019;80:e9–e10.

10. Gupta L. Growing up Hindu and Muslim: how early does it happen? Econ Polit Wkly. 2008;43:35–41.

11. Chatterjee R, Gupta B, Bose S. Oral screening for pre-cancerous lesions among areca-nut chewing population from rural India. Oral Health Prev Dent. 2015;13:509–14.

12. Prabhu RV, Prabhu V, Chatra L, Shenai P, Suvarna N, Dandekeri S. Areca nut and its role in oral submucous fibrosis. J Clin Exp Dent. 2014;6:569–75.

13. Kiran G, Muni Sekhar M, Hunasgi S, Ahmed SA, Suri C, Krishna A. Plasma fibrinogen degradation products in betel nut chewers – with and without oral submucous fibrosis. J Oral Maxillofac Pathol. 2013;17:324–8.

14. Mathew P, Austin RD, Varghese SS, Manojkumar. Estimation and comparison of copper content in raw areca nuts and commercial areca nut products: implications in increasing prevalence of oral submucous fibrosis (OSMF). J Clin Diagn Res. 2014;8:247–9.

15. Mohammed F, Manohar V, Jose M, et al. Estimation of copper in saliva and areca nut products and its correlation with histological grades of oral submucous fibrosis. J Oral Pathol Med. 2015;44:208–13.

16. Khan I, Pant I, Narra S, et al. Epithelial atrophy in oral submucous fibrosis is mediated by copper (II) and arecoline of areca nut. J Cell Mol Med. 2015;19:2397–412.

17. Hosein M, Mohiuddin S, Fatima N. Association between grading of oral submucous fibrosis with frequency and consumption of areca nut and its derivatives in a wide age group: a multi-centric cross sectional study from Karachi, Pakistan. J Cancer Prev. 2015;20:216–22.

18. Prasad S, Anand R, Dhingra C. Betel nut chewing behavior and its association with oral mucosal lesions and conditions in Ghaziabad, India. Oral Health Prev Dent. 2014;12:241–8.
19. Anand R, Dhingra C, Prasad S, Menon I. Betel nut chewing and its deleterious effects on oral cavity. J Cancer Res Ther. 2014;10:499–505.
20. Yanduri S, Kumar VB, Suma S, Madhura MG. Lichenoid features and fibrosis: coexistence in quid-induced oral lesions. J Contemp Dent Pract. 2015;16:389–93.
21. Abdul Khader NF, Dyasanoor S. Assessment of salivary flow rate and pH among areca nut chewers and oral submucous fibrosis subjects: a comparative study. J Cancer Prev. 2015;20:208–15.
22. Moss J, Kawamoto C, Pokhrel P, Paulino Y, Herzog T. Developing a betel quid cessation program on the island of Guam. Pac Asia Inq. 2015;6:144–50.
23. Liu B, Shen M, Xiong J, et al. Synergistic effects of betel quid chewing, tobacco use (in the form of cigarette smoking), and alcohol consumption on the risk of malignant transformation of oral submucous fibrosis (OSF): a case-control study in Hunan Province, China. Oral Surg Oral Med Oral Pathol Oral Radiol. 2015;120:337–45.
24. Abanmi AA, Al Zouman AY, Alhussaini H, Al-Asmari A. Prayer marks. Int J Dermatol. 2002;41:411–4.
25. Bowen J. Salat in Indonesia: the social meanings of an Islamic ritual. Man (NS). 1989;24:600–19.
26. Barankin B. Prayer marks. Int J Dermatol. 2004;43:985–6.
27. Orenay OM, Sarifakioglu E. Prayer mark on the forehead: hyperpigmentation. Ann Dermatol. 2015;27:107–8.
28. ur Rehman H, Asfour NA. Clinical images: prayer nodules. CMAJ. 2010;182:19.
29. Sharma V, Sharma A, Aggarwal S. Prayer-marks heralding acute coronary syndrome. J Health Popul Nutr. 2011;29:660.
30. Cangiano M, Chisti MJ, Pietroni MA, Smith JH. Extending prayer marks as a sign of worsening chronic disease. J Health Popul Nutr. 2011;29:290–1.
31. Mishriki YY. Skin commotion from repetitive devotion. Prayer callus. Postgrad Med. 1999;105:153–4.
32. El-Din Anbar T, Abdel-Rahman AT, El-Khayyat MA, El-Azhary AE. Vitiligo on anterior aspect of neck in Muslim females: case series. Int J Dermatol. 2008;47:178–9.
33. Ghislain PD, Dinet Y, Delescluse J. Orf contamination may occur during religious events. J Am Acad Dermatol. 2000;42:848.

34. Malik M, Bharier M, Tahan S. Orf acquired during religious observance. Arch Dermatol. 2009;145:606–8.
35. Nougairede A, Fossati C, Salez N, Cohen-Bacrie S, Ninove L, Michel F, Aboukais S, Buttner M, Zandotti C, de Lamballerie X, Charrel RN. Sheep-to-human transmission of Orf virus during eid al-adha religious practices, France. Emerg Infect Dis. 2013;19:102–5.
36. Veraldi S, Nazzaro G, Varia F, Cuka E. Presentation of orf (ecthyma contagiosum) after sheep slaughtering for religious feasts. Infection. 2014;42:767–9.
37. James J, Saladi RN, Fox JL. Traction alopecia in Sikh male patients. J Am Board Fam Med. 2007;20:497–8.
38. Karimaian-Teherani D, El Shabrawi-Caelen L, Tanew A. Traction alopecia in two adolescent Sikh brothers-an underrecognized problem unmasked by migration. Pediatr Dermatol. 2011;28:336–8.
39. Kanwar AJ, Kaur S, Basak P, Sharma R. Traction alopecia in Sikh males. Arch Dermatol. 1989;125:1587.
40. Williams HC. Turban ear. Arch Dermatol. 1994;130:117–9.
41. Mansouri Y, Orpin SD. Are these real turban tumours? Clin Exp Dermatol. 2013;38:424–5.
42. Naimer SA, Trattner A, Biton A, Avinoach I, Vardy D. Davener's dermatosis: a variant of friction hypermelanosis. J Am Acad Dermatol. 2000;42:442–5.
43. Cho S, Lee SJ, Lee JH, Cho SB. Treatment of Davener's dermatosis using a 1064-nm Q-switched Nd:YAG laser with low fluence. Int J Dermatol. 2012;51:1394–6.
44. Gilead L, Vardy DA, Schamroth J. Tefillin dermatitis (a phylacteric phenomenon). J Am Acad Dermatol. 1995;32:812–3.
45. Trattner A, David M. Tefillin dermatitis. J Am Acad Dermatol. 2005;52:831–3.
46. Friedmann AC, Goldsmith P. Tefillin contact dermatitis: a problem in the devout. Contact Dermatitis. 2008;59:188–9.
47. Feit NE, Weinberg JM, DeLeo VA. Cutaneous disease and religious practice: case of allergic contact dermatitis to tefillin and review of the literature. Int J Dermatol. 2004;43:886–8.
48. Ross B, Brancaccio RR. Allergic contact dermatitis to tefillin. J Am Acad Dermatol. 1996;34:152–3.
49. Goldammer KMA. Religious symbolism and iconography. Britannica Website. 2010.
50. Goodheart HP. "Devotional dermatoses": a new nosologic entity? J Am Acad Dermatol. 2001;44:543.

51. Sanchez MR. Cutaneous diseases in Latinos. Dermatol Clin. 2003;21:689–97.
52. Lopez EA. Modern Spain. ABC-CLIO, LLC: Santa Barbara; 2016.
53. Camacho F. Acquired circumscribed hypertrichosis in the 'costaleros' who bear the 'pasos' during Holy Week in Seville, Spain. Arch Dermatol. 1995;131:361–3.

Chapter 5
Environmental Dermatoses

Nicole Trepanowski, Nicole Patzelt, and Neelam A. Vashi

A variety of region-specific practices have been created by certain cultures to adapt to their unique environments. In some cases, these practices can lead to the development of dermatoses. In this chapter, we will discuss four of these environmental dermatoses: mudi-chood, Kangri cancer, fissured plantar keratoderma, and Ladakh dermatoses. It is important for dermatologists to consider these dermatoses

N. Trepanowski
Boston University School of Medicine, Boston, MA, USA

N. Patzelt
Department of Dermatology, Boston Medical Center, Boston, MA, USA

N. A. Vashi (✉)
Boston University School of Medicine, Boston, MA, USA

Department of Dermatology, Boston Medical Center, Boston, MA, USA

Department of Dermatology, Boston University Center for Ethnic Skin, Boston, MA, USA

Boston University Cosmetic and Laser Center, Boston, MA, USA

Department of Veteran Affairs, Boston Health Care System, Boston, MA, USA

© The Author(s) 2021   107
N. A. Vashi (ed.), *Cultural Practices and Dermatoses*,
https://doi.org/10.1007/978-3-030-68992-6_5

when treating patients from these geographical areas, as management may differ from otherwise common disorders.

The following conditions draw from published case reports and series on environmental practices that lead to dermatologic complications. A paucity of published data and formal studies on environmental dermatoses limit conclusions regarding prevalence of these conditions.

This chapter is divided into subsections based on the dermatologic condition described. Information on the background, complications, and treatment of each entity is provided. Table 5.1 provides a summary of this information.

Mudi-chood

Background

Mudi-chood (also discussed in Chap. 3) was first described by Sugathan et al. in 1972 in the state of Kerala in southern India [1, 2]. The term derives from the Malayalam language and translates to "heat of the hair" [3]. Women in the state of Kerala commonly wash and oil their long hair and leave it to dry in the sun. Coconut or sesame oil are traditionally used, and the long hair is tied into knots at the ends [1]. Herbal products are often added to the hair oils [4]. The damp environment and high temperatures lead to sweating and a follicular reaction on areas of skin that are in contact with the hair [5, 6]. An increased incidence of mudi-chood has been noted in the summer months of Western India, supporting the fact that heat is likely a contributing factor [4]. Although most commonly seen in young women, Pillai et al. describes one case of mudi-chood in a man [6, 7].

Complications

Mudi-chood has been reported on the upper back, forearm, neck, and pinnae [6]. Adverse events associated with mudi-chood include pruritic and pigmented lichenoid dermatitis

TABLE 5.1 Summary of environmental dermatoses

Country of origin	Name of dermatoses	Mechanism/ Definition	Dermatologic complications	Prevention	Treatment
Southern India (Kerala)	Mudi-chood	Applying oils to long hair in a hot and humid environment causes friction and follicular reaction [4–6]	Pruritic, pigmented lichenoid dermatitis with follicular, flat-topped papules with scale on the upper back, forearm, neck, and pinnae [5, 6]	Short hair, regular washing with shampoo [6]	3–5% salicylic acid +/– topical corticosteroids [1]
Kashmir valley of India	Kangri cancer	A kangri is a clay pot that contains coal embers that is tucked between the legs and abdomen to provide warmth [8–11]	Erythema ab igne, Bowen's disease, squamous cell carcinoma, burns [8, 9, 13]	Alternate methods of heat conservation	Wide local excision, ± radiation, chemotherapy, Mohs surgery, cryotherapy, targeted therapy, photodynamic or light therapy, scraping, or dermabrasion [11, 16, 17]
Congo Brazzaville (the Republic of the Congo)	Fissured plantar keratoderma	Unknown origin, but proposed to be due to poor hygiene or leprosy [18]	Fissured plantar keratoderma [18]	Treat underlying cause [19]	Keratolytics, emollients, PUVA therapy, balneotherapy [18]

with follicular, flat-topped papules and scale [5, 6]. Papules have a thin keratin rim with a depression in the center and may become confluent [6]. Koebner's phenomenon has been noted [6]. Typical histopathologic exam of lesions shows irregular acanthosis, hyperkeratosis with intervening layers of parakeratosis, edema of the dermal papillae, decreased melanin in the basal layers, and mild infiltration with chronic inflammatory cells in the upper dermis [1]. Occasional suprapapillary thinning has been noted, and capillaries may be dilated [6]. Spongiosis and lymphocytic exocytosis have also been reported [5].

Treatment

Mudi-chood can be prevented by maintaining short hair and regular washing with shampoo [1, 6]. Mudi-chood can be treated with 3–5% salicylic acid [1]. Topical corticosteroids may be added to the treatment [1].

Kangri Cancer

Background

Kangri cancer is a heat induced squamous cell carcinoma that arises from preexisting lesions of erythema ab igne, followed with progression to Bowen's disease and squamous cell carcinoma [8, 9]. A Kangri is a fire pot tucked between the inner thighs and abdomen to generate warmth [9]. It is an earthenware clay pot with an outer encasement of wicker [8, 10]. The inside of the pot is traditionally filled with coal [8]. A Kangri is typically 6 inches in diameter [9]. Kangri is traditionally carried under one's phiran or pheran, the Kashmiri cloak. If a person is wearing a jacket, it may be used as a hand warmer [9]. Heat may be provided by a Kangri for up to 9 hours and temperatures can reach up to 150 °F [9, 11]. Kangri are traditionally used in the Kashmir Valley of India, the northern-most and coldest part of India [9]. They are sometimes given as wedding gifts [12]. Kangri serve as a popular method of heat conservation during winter in the Kashmir Valley because they are portable and inexpensive [11].

Complications

Kangri cancer typically affects the anatomical areas that come into close contact with the Kangri, predominantly the inner thighs, lower abdomen, legs, and feet [8, 10–12]. Typically, a progression is noted from erythema ab igne to Bowen's disease to squamous cell carcinoma. Kangri cancer usually begins as a papular skin growth over erythema ab igne. The most common presentation is a nodulo-ulcerative growth with a history of pain and bleeding [9]. Kangri has also been associated with burns in epileptic patients [13].

Prolonged exposure to heat is frequently associated with the development of Kangri cancer. Products of combustion from the coals like tar from chinar leaves, wood ash, and volatile substances may play a secondary role [12, 14, 15].

Kangri cancer has been reported in both males and females although studies disagree whether the incidence is higher in one gender [12, 14, 16]. Kangri cancer is predominantly seen in persons older than 50 years suggesting that prolonged use is necessary for squamous cell transformation [8].

Discontinuation of Kangri may lead to spontaneous resolution in most cases, but prolonged use results in ulceration and malignant transformation [10, 14, 16]. Ulceration occurs in greater than 70% of cases [16]. Squamous cell carcinoma that arises due to Kangri tends to be aggressive with 30–50% of cases experiencing locoregional metastases [16]. A higher incidence of parasitic infection and resultant anemia in the Kashmir Valley may contribute to the aggressive behavior of this cancer [10].

Treatment

Wide surgical excision and removal of the entire tumor is the preferred method of treatment for Kangri cancer. This may be followed by radiation therapy and/or chemotherapy if deemed appropriate. In some instances, other methods of treatment including targeted therapy, photodynamic light or laser therapy, scraping and dermabrasion, Mohs surgery, and cryotherapy have been used [11]. The use of 55–65 Gy adjuvant radiotherapy after wide local excision has been associated with positive outcomes in patients with positive resection lines, perineural or perivascular infiltration, and locoregional occurrence [16]. External beam radiotherapy has been shown to successfully treat local recurrence of Kangri cancer [17].

Fissured Plantar Keratoderma

Background

Fissured plantar keratoderma has been reported among the female Bantu population of Congo Brazzaville (the Republic of the Congo) [18].

Complications

It is unclear as to why women in this population are experiencing fissured plantar keratoderma, but poor hygiene and leprosy have been suggested as potential causes [18]. Plantar keratoderma can be hereditary or acquired, and some etiologies of acquired forms include environmental, chemical, drug-induced, immunologic, paraneoplastic, nutritional, infectious, aquagenic and idiopathic [19].

Women with fissured plantar keratoderma in the Bantu population of Congo Brazzaville experience divorce, forced celibacy, and public humiliation from clan and marital partners due to their condition [18].

Treatment

Topical keratolytics, emollients, PUVA therapy, and balneotherapy have been suggested as possible treatments for this population [18]. In addition, treating the underlying cause, if one can be identified, is an important treatment consideration [19].

Conclusion

In this chapter, we have discussed various dermatoses specific to certain environments. Many of these environmental dermatoses are only diagnosed after taking a thorough history, as their presentation can be similar to other more common conditions. It is important for physicians to consider the role of the environment in the development of dermatoses, as managment may differ depending on the cause of a patient's condition.

Patients may be unaware of the role that the environment or their practices may play in the development of their dermatologic conditions. It is important for the physician to work with the patient to develop the best treatment plan for that individual patient.

References

1. Sugathan P. Mudi-chood disease. Dermatol Online J. 1999;5(2):5.
2. Kuruvila S, Ganguly S. Mudi-chood outside Kerala. Indian J Dermatol. 2013;58(3):246.
3. Gupta G, Reshme P, Raju K, et al. Mudichood: well-known but rare entity. Int J Trichol. 2013;5(2):101.
4. Gharpuray MB, Kulkarni V, Tolat S. Mudi-chood: an unusual tropical dermatosis. Int J Dermatol. 1992;31(6):396–7.
5. Kumar D, Kuruvila M, Upadya GM, Kumar P, Nirupama M. Novel dermoscopic findings in mudi-chood disease – a case report. Int J Dermatol. 2017;56(7):776–8.
6. Gupta D, Thappa DM. Dermatoses due to Indian cultural practices. Indian J Dermatol. 2015;60(1):3–12.

7. Sugathan P, Martin AM. Mudi-chood: on the forearm. Indian J Dermatol. 2011;56(2):228–9. https://doi.org/10.4103/0019-5154.80430.

8. Wani I. Kangri cancer. Surgery. 2010;147(4):586–8.

9. Hassan I, Sajad P. Kangri: a boon or bane for Kashmiris. Indian Dermatol Online J. 2016;7(6):551–3.

10. Suryanarayan CR. Kangri cancer in Kashmir valley: preliminary study. J Surg Oncol. 1973;5(4):327–33.

11. Sharma H, Rajeshwari, Sahu U, Kumar G, Kaur CD. A spectrum of skin cancer in Kashmir valley of India: kangri cancer. J Atoms Molecules. 2019;9(1):1196–205.

12. Neve EF. Squamous celled epithelioma due to kangri burn. Natl Med J India. 2010;23(1):51–3, 48, 54–5.

13. Baba PF, Sharma S, Wani A. Epileptic burn injuries in Kashmir valley: is 'Kangri' a boon or bane? Indian J Burns. 2019;27(1):95.

14. Hassan I, Sajad P, Reshi R. Histopathological analysis of the cutaneous changes due to kangri use in Kashmiri population: a hospital based study. Indian J Dermatol. 2013;58(3):188–90.

15. Bajaj AK, Pandey RK, Misra K, et al. Contact depigmentation caused by an azo dye in alta. Contact Dermatitis. 1998;38(4):189–93.

16. Teli MA, Khan NA, Darzi MA, et al. Recurrence pattern in squamous cell carcinoma of skin of lower extremities and abdominal wall (Kangri cancer) in Kashmir valley of Indian subcontinent: impact of various treatment modalities. Indian J Dermatol. 2009;54(4):342–6.

17. Teli M, Darzi M, Gupta M, et al. Recurrent Kangri cancer treated with external beam radiotherapy on a cobalt unit. Indian J Cancer. 2008;45(3):134–5.

18. Lenga-Loumingou IA. Dermatoses and traditions: fissured plantar keratoderma, a discriminating factor in bantu society in the Congo Brazzaville. Int J Womens Dermatol. 2020;6(2):125–6.

19. Patel S, Zirwas M, English JC. Acquired palmoplantar keratoderma. Am J Clin Dermatol. 2007;8(1):1–11.

Chapter 6
Cultural Competency

Neda So and Michelle Rodrigues

What Is Cultural Competency?

Culture and Health Beliefs

Culture is a broad and dynamic term, referring to the coherent set of characteristics (such as beliefs, values, customs and behaviours) of individuals, communities and the broader socio-political context to which they identify.

Groups may be collectively distinct in terms of the following dimensions: demographic factors (e.g. age, gender, sexual orientation, ethnic/racial identities, immigration status, abilities), beliefs (e.g. religion or spirituality), location (e.g. country, region, district), time periods (e.g. decades, centuries), social context (e.g. school, workplace, occupation, social clubs, political groups, governments) and socioeconomic position (e.g. social class, literacy level, education level, income/finances, occupation, marital status, parenthood).

The features that make them distinct can include a range of concrete, behavioural and abstract characteristics, as shown in Table 6.1 [1].

N. So · M. Rodrigues (✉)
Royal Children's Hospital, Melbourne, VIC, Australia

Chroma Dermatology, Melbourne, VIC, Australia

© The Author(s) 2021
N. A. Vashi (ed.), *Cultural Practices and Dermatoses*,
https://doi.org/10.1007/978-3-030-68992-6_6

TABLE 6.1 Nitza Hidalgo's three levels of culture

Level	Description	Characteristics
1. The concrete	The most visible, surface-level dimensions of culture	Dress, music, food, games, language
2. The behavioural	The expression of one's values and how one belongs to their external social structure	Social roles, gender roles, family structures, institutions, political affiliations, relationships, languages, non-verbal communication
3. The symbolic	The abstract intellectual concepts defining or shared by the culture	Beliefs, ideas, assumptions, worldviews, values, rituals, traditions, customs, spirituality, religion

Data from Hidalgo [1]

The concept of culture is constantly evolving in response to the forces of globalization, immigration and diversification. It is important to recognise that patients are individuals formed from the unique circumstances and experiences of their lives.

It is from their cultural heritage that an individual develops the foundations of their attitudes and behaviours towards health practitioners and the medical institution. Culture influences patients' help-seeking behaviour, including which health practitioner is first approached, duration between symptom onset and consult, treatment preferences, and expectations for healing.

Multiculturally Competent Healthcare

Multiculturalism refers to the diversity among populations in cultural dimensions, such as race, language, religion, and socioeconomic position [2]. It is founded on the premise that different cultures can co-exist peacefully and equitably in the same society, with respect for each other's unique characteristics and for the value of diversity to society. The ethos of multiculturalism calls for inclusiveness and the integration of different cultural components into the same social fabric.

Cultural competency is defined as the "ongoing capacity of healthcare systems, organizations, and professionals to provide for diverse patient populations high-quality care that is safe, patient and family centred, evidence based, and equitable" [3]. *Cross-cultural communication* in healthcare is the application of values of cultural competency in facilitating effective communication between practitioners and patients.

Providing *multiculturally competent healthcare* refers to delivering patient-centred care in a way that is respectful of and aligned with the patient's cultural health beliefs, practices and value systems. They are provided in congruence with patients' preferred mode of communication – including language fluency, level of health literacy, communication needs and health values. At a "culturally and linguistically appropriate service", a patient should receive this level of care at every interaction with each staff member.

Why Is Cultural Competency Important and How Does It Relate to Outcomes?

Multiculturalism and diversity are increasing within societies globally. In the United States, minority populations currently comprise an estimated third of the population, however, are projected to cross-over to becoming a "minority-majority" nation with over 50% of the population consisting of "minority groups" by 2050, due to factors such as ageing, population growth and immigration [4].

However, health disparities nonetheless persist for patients from minority groups. Health disparities (or health inequities) refer to the differences in epidemiological measures of health (such as incidence, prevalence, morbidity, mortality and burden of disease) that adversely affect groups of people who lack political, social or economic power, often as a result of historical and systemic discrimination and injustices experienced by their cultural group [5–7]. These vulnerable groups include immigrants, refugees, marginalised people, and racial and ethnic monitory groups, who generally have poorer quality health outcomes than the majority population.

Through understanding the gaps that exist, we as healthcare professionals can strive towards treating everyone equitably – not simply equally, but *fairly* in accordance with their circumstances.

Patient-Doctor Relationship

Differences between the clinician and patient's cultural background can subconsciously impact the delivery of quality patient care. As a practitioner, being cognisant of methods to enhance cross-cultural communication increases one's skill set and confidence in treating diverse communities. Good cross-cultural communication gives patients a greater sense of comfort and rapport, increases the likelihood of compliance and empowers patients in the healthcare setting.

Dermatology

Cultural competency is especially important in the field of dermatology as it is a mostly external specialty that focuses on conditions of heavily culture-laden features such as skin and hair. Patients from different cultural groups are likely to have a different epidemiology of dermatological issues as discussed in this text, which should be addressed uniquely with patients – for example, skin of colour responds differently to factors such as the sun (greater hyperpigmentation – see Fig. 6.1) and the scarring process (risk of keloid scarring – see Fig. 6.2).

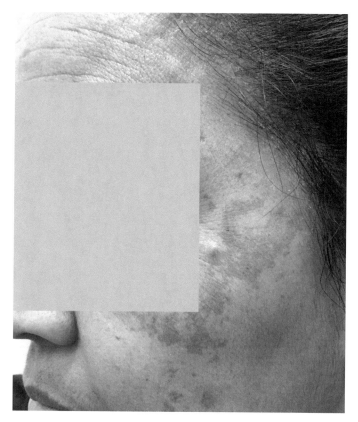

FIGURE 6.1 Facial melasma in a patient with darker skin. (Courtesy of Dr Michelle Rodrigues)

Barriers

There are several barriers that patients may face in obtaining culturally competent health care. There may be *systemic or structural barriers* of an ecological nature that are related to the social determinants of health, including access to housing, food, transportation, education, employment and recreation.

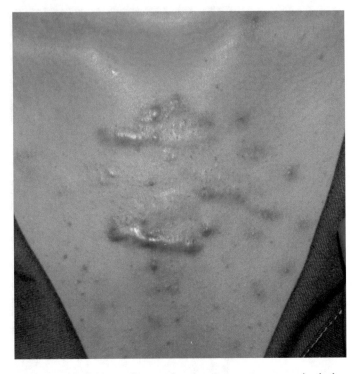

FIGURE 6.2 Keloid scarring on the chest – more common in darker skin types. (Courtesy of Dr Michelle Rodrigues)

There is often also a lack of targeted public health education for people of different cultural backgrounds. Preventative health campaigns for skin cancer awareness need to be tailored to individual cultural groups. For those with African skin, for example, skin cancer awareness programs need to focus on acral melanomas, melanomas of the nail and risk factors for other types of skin cancers more prevalent in this group of patients.

Language barriers also pose a significant barrier to equitable access of healthcare for diverse patients and may contribute to or exacerbate low *health literacy*, which refers to a patient's capacity to "obtain, process and understand basic health information and services needed to make appropriate health decisions" [8–10]. When patients have poorer health literacy, they are less likely to ask questions and express concerns, and may encounter barriers to understanding medical decisions and treatment plans – including the benefits, common side effects, mechanism of action of medications [11].

How to Improve Competency?

Educating Health Care Providers

One of the barriers in achieving cultural competency is the widespread lack of appropriate cultural competency training for health care professionals. An effective curriculum should be interspersed throughout all the years of medical training and incorporated as ongoing professional development.

Theoretical teaching should be combined with case-based practical learning simulating real-life scenarios, such as role-plays with patient actors. Students and trainees should be exposed to a range of clinical scenarios from a diverse patient base with different cultural and social backgrounds that reflect the cultural composition of their local community.

Diversifying the Clinician Workforce

Ethnically diverse populations remain under-represented minorities among the clinician workforce [12]. For example, in the United States, only 5.8% of physicians identify as being of African American ancestry compared to 12% of the population, and 4.4% of physicians identify as being of Hispanic ancestry compared to 17.8% of the population [13, 14]. In dermatology, the representation is lower, with 4.2% identifying as of Hispanic ancestry, and 3% identifying as African American [13, 15].

Steps such as prioritising diversity in recruitment, offering mentorship and exposing potential applicants to specialties with less diverse representation, may improve cultural competency and accessibility of dermatology as a field [13].

The Clinician Mindset

An initial step in developing cultural competency is in *self-reflection* and exploration of one's own cultural identity. We must become self-aware of our own cultural background and the inherent assumptions we hold in our worldview. Through this understanding, we may be able to examine our personal and cultural biases and understand how they may differ from those of our patients.

Self-Directed Learning

We may then be able to embark on *self-directed learning* to understand common sets of cultural health beliefs and preferences and gain familiarity with the range of traditional healing therapies or practices used by various cultural groups.

Greater cultural competency may be developed with time, experience and exposure. The more practice a clinician has interacting with patients from a cultural group, the greater the opportunity to gain a deeper understanding of the pre-existing health beliefs, issues and values important to that group.

Collaborate with Community

In order to coordinate optimal patient care, a multidisciplinary team approach is often used. When treating patients from a diverse cultural background, it is even more important to reach out to community health experts (for example, Aboriginal Liaison Officers in Australia), or social workers, case managers, and pastoral care to assist in integrating a patient's care journey with their cultural background.

Communicating Effectively

The clinician should be striving towards a goal of achieving effective interpersonal communication with the patient, with a mindset of being open, non-judgemental, and aiming to provide a safe space for patients to feel comfortable divulging more sensitive thoughts. Should they disclose any concerns, these feelings should be validated and reaffirmed.

The clinician should facilitate specific requests such as the participation of family and accommodate as much as possible any other specific cultural requests. There should also be some flexibility in one's interviewing style to adapt it to patients of different cultural backgrounds. For example, some may feel intimidated by direct eye contact and prefer an averted gaze, and patients who do not yet have a strong rapport with the practitioner may prefer to avoid taboo or sensitive topics.

Understanding Patient Approaches to Doctors

Some cultures may have a baseline mistrust or suspicion of doctors practicing "Western" medical or surgical treatments, sometimes originating from a history of racial discrimination and segregation [16].

Yet other cultures tend to view clinicians as authority figures, wherein doctors tend to practice a more paternalistic communication style, with less shared decision making [17]. Out of respect to the doctor's expert opinion, patients may be reluctant to share their health beliefs or question doctors' recommendations [18].

Contrarily, some cultures value highly a more informal, personal clinician-patient relationship (such as the Hispanic concept of *personalismo,* the personal relationship [19], and may expect that a professional relationship may develop a more personal dimension over time. This can involve sitting in closer proximity, or providing reassuring gestures such as a hand on the shoulder [19]. Physicians who resist this can be at risk of being seen as impersonal or disinterested, which may alienate the patient or decrease treatment compliance.

Understanding Patients' Health Beliefs and Models of Illness

Some individuals have alternative or unconventional beliefs about the causes of certain pathologies, not necessarily specific to any culture or religion. For example, some believe illness to be a result of an imbalance between opposing energies (such as the Chinese philosophy of yin and yang), or attach beliefs to foods as having opposing qualities such as "hot" or "cold", or hold a strong focus on the ability of food to cause or cure disease.

In some religions, illness is perceived as a natural progression along the course of life. Yet others believe in pre-determination or fatalism (Hispanic *fatalismo*) and viewing illness as the result of supernatural intervention, bad karma, social dysfunction, or failure to fulfil their expected moral or religious duties [20, 21]. Individuals with fatalistic beliefs may be less proactive in seeking treatment, especially if circumstances are complicated by other barriers such as financial or logistical restrictions. Alternatively, they may continue to participate in detrimental health behaviours with limited belief in their ability to achieve positive health change.

It is imperative that health professionals respectfully explore and address these beliefs with patients. These beliefs may be corrected with a biological or mechanistic explanation should the patient be open to receiving it.

Traditional Medicine (TM) and Complementary and Alternative Medicines (CAM)

The World Health Organisation defines traditional medicine as "including diverse health practices, approaches, knowledge and beliefs incorporating plant, animal and/or mineral based medicines, spiritual therapies, manual techniques and exercises, applied singularly or in combination to maintain well-being, as well as to treat, diagnose or prevent illness" [22, 23].

Many cultures place a lot of trust in traditional healers, who have a holistic approach to illness and often share the patient's cultural views [20]. Those who use traditional medicines or folk health practices often believe that these "natural" remedies are safer than pharmaceutical treatment or operative management. There is a limited body of evidence supporting the efficacy of traditional and complementary medicines over biomedical therapies. Furthermore, "natural" does not equate to "harmless", and these may likewise carry risks of adverse events or drug interactions.

Some may choose to seek traditional practitioners or therapy in substitution or to or in combination with prescription medication. This could be due to a variety of reasons including fear of side effects, confusion, the appearance or size of tablets, and not considering the possibility of drug interactions. Using multiple therapies may introduce risks of non-compliance, drug interactions and side effects.

Clinicians should be able to discuss traditional medicines with patients in an open, respectful, non-judgemental and interested manner to encourage patient trust [24]. If it is detected on history that a patient is using traditional medication, ask the patient to take a photograph or bring in the remedy to investigate and discuss together. If the traditional or complementary medicine is deemed to be harmless or have a positive placebo effect, they could be carefully integrated into a patients' healthcare plan to promote adherence and provide a holistic and culturally supportive approach.

Assessing Language Barriers

Clinicians may use objective assessments, such as the Test of Functional Health Literacy in Adults (TOFHLA) [25] to rapidly estimate the patient's ability to read and understand common medical terms. An objective assessment is more reliable than a clinician's estimation, which may be based on assumptions or stereotypes.

Should the clinician determine that the patient has language barriers, strategies for the clinician to overcome these barriers include speaking clearly and slowly, use lay terms and avoiding a patronising or condescending tone. The clinician should also take care to explain information using photos or diagrams and should write down medical terms for patients' reference.

Patient Education Material

Interpretation refers to the "process of understanding and analysing a spoken or signed message and re-expressing that message faithfully, accurately, and objectively in another language, taking the cultural and social context into account" [26]. The role of the interpreter extends beyond converting one language into another. Interpretation encompasses the nuances of culture, idioms, family dynamics, non-verbal cues and possible underlying explanatory model for illness.

When seeing patients with limited English proficiency, it is important that a certified medical interpreter be used to facilitate medical discussions, as they are often high-stakes discussions with potentially serious adverse consequences. In a hospital setting it may be possible to organise an in-house interpreter in advance, especially in advance of an outpatient clinic or a ward round. Attempt to meet briefly with the interpreter before the consultation to discuss the goals of the discussion, especially if the issues are complex.

The optimal physical arrangement is positioning the physician and patient so that they are facing and speaking to each other directly, with the interpreter sitting beside the patient. An alternative and more natural position is a triangular arrangement with balanced space and symbolic power in the conversation.

Economic constraints, time limitations in busy clinical settings, or limited availability after hours can contribute to under-utilisation of qualified interpreters, leading to using ad hoc interpreters or attempting to manage without. However, "ad hoc" interpreting with family members can be problematic as they may be unfamiliar with medical terminology, or provide abridged or biased recounts with an overlay of their own opinion [27]. If interpreters are unavailable, in-person interpreters may be accessed via other modalities such as telephone services or remote video interpreting.

While using an interpreter will overcome most language barriers, it does not overcome barriers of physician cultural competency or any social barriers. A dual approach must be used.

The Cultural Interview

There are multiple approaches to the cultural interview described to elicit a patient's cultural context. These are generally a series of open-ended questions that can be used as an interview tool by the clinician upon diagnosis to explore a patient's explanatory model for illness. Through a series of directed questions, the aim is to elicit how a patient understands the illness, identify any preconceived thoughts, and elucidate any fears or concerns.

The Kleinman 'Explanatory Models Approach' [28] and the DSM-V Cultural Formulation Interview [29] outline a model of interviewing that can be adapted for your clinical context. The standard questions are open-ended and exploratory, and generally applicable to most patients.

The Medical Consultation

Elicit the Patient's Health Beliefs and Explanatory Model of Illness

It is important to understand how the patient perceives their illness, the predisposing factors and the psychosocial ramifications (Fig. 6.3). This is particularly relevant for vulnerable groups who are at risk of non-compliance, or patients of culturally and linguistically diverse backgrounds who are about to receive a new diagnosis of a chronic condition that requires extensive and careful management, with significant

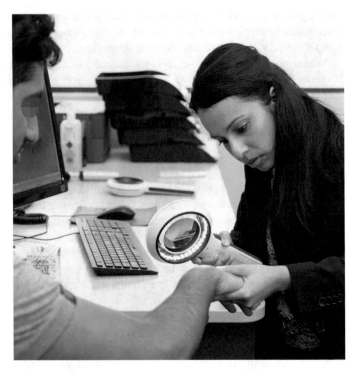

FIGURE 6.3 A dermatological medical consultation. (Courtesy of Dr Michelle Rodrigues)

morbidity or risk of disability. It may be difficult to convey the notion of acute versus chronic illness, and the difference between curing, managing and preventing disease in your management plan.

The negative feelings surrounding the illness may not have simple biomedical explanations. Rather, they may be associated with perceived moral failings, life challenges, or conflict with loved ones. It is important to attempt to recognise any fears, identify their source, gently correct any underlying misconceptions, address patients' cultural beliefs and values, and offer reassurance. A gentle slow approach may also assist in eliciting any harmful or risky behaviours.

Breaking Bad News

There is variability in the level of information patients wish to receive – some would prefer that confronting news be omitted, and others prefer to know as much detail as possible. It is important to question patients and family thoroughly to gauge their preferences regarding receiving diagnoses, and subsequently adopt a more flexible approach to delivering bad news. When breaking bad news or giving a diagnosis, it is useful to approach the diagnosis with a clear biomedical approach. The diagnosis should be given a specific name or label, and the pathophysiology explained in a factual way to minimise any feelings of shame or beliefs that the cause stems from personal failures. The SPIKES model, a six-step protocol can then be used to gently deliver bad news: Setting, Perception, Invitation, Knowledge, Emotions/Empathy, Strategy/Summary [30].

Treatment Decision-Making

Some patients desire full autonomy over all medical decisions, and others prefer to articulate preferences but leave the final decision in the hands of the doctor as the medical expert. Assess how the patient wishes to make medical decisions and consider potential preferences for shared decision making with family involvement or a medical power of attorney.

Patient Education

Aim to ensure that the patient understands as much as they are able about their disease state, and treatment options, with consideration for cultural influences and in congruence with their level of health literacy. Explain the illness aetiology, course, treatment, indication(s), rationale, risks, benefits, alternatives, and common and important adverse effects. Discuss the advantages and disadvantages of each modality of investigation or treatment. Importantly, emphasise to patients that they have a choice, that some options may carry divided expert opinion, or that investigations are imperfect with false positives and negatives. It is important to check the patient's understanding by asking a combination of open-ended questions (for example, "tell me what you understand about your condition"), and close-ended questions (for example, "when should your medication be taken?") to identify any gaps in understanding and to reinforce knowledge.

Gently probe to elicit any trepidation a patient may display to explore potential underlying fears (e.g. radiotherapy, medication-related, procedural) and attempt to offer reassurance by giving accurate clinical details. Provide opportunities for the patient to express concerns or health beliefs, ask for more information, or express treatment preferences. Be aware that excessive brevity may override a patient's perception of autonomy, and conversely, providing too much information or pushing for a final treatment decision may overwhelm or alienate them.

Shared or Participatory Decision-Making

Many medical decisions are unilateral, made by clinicians with limited input from patients or their families. However, in shared decision making, patients and clinicians can collaborate to weigh the risks and benefits of medical decisions against patient's preferences and values. Together, they can negotiate medical plans with the aim of improving patient satisfaction, compliance, and ultimately, creating better health outcomes. Some patients will desire full autonomy over all medical decisions, and others prefer to articulate preferences but leave the final decision in the hands of the doctor as the medical expert. Assess how the patient wishes to make medical decisions and consider such preferences for shared decision making. This may include involvement of family or a medical power of attorney.

Furthermore, cultural competency can be instrumental to practicing evidence-based medicine, avoiding defensive medicine and minimising overuse or misuse of clinical services or treatments. A clinician who can delve deeper into the beliefs, values and fears that underlie patient requests for over-investigation or over-treatment is better able to readjust patient expectations and provide reassurance while maintaining patient engagement.

After a treatment plan has been jointly decided, clinicians should provide patients with an overview of what to expect when navigating their management, follow up plans and any hospital systems. The bureaucracy of health networks can be unfamiliar and intimidating, especially for vulnerable patients. Clinicians may also act as a "*cultural broker*" or interpreter of biomedicine and health systems, using explanations to increase the accessibility of healthcare to patients.

The LEARN model is a framework for cross-cultural communication that summarises the above steps and enhances shared decision making. The acronym stands for: *Listen* to patients' perspectives, *Explain* medical views, *Acknowledge* similarities and differences, *Recommend* a course of action, *Negotiate* plans [31].

Conclusion

With growing diversity, it is increasingly important that the global health workforce is equipped to care for patients from diverse cultural backgrounds. Through empathy and thoughtfulness, all practitioners can strive towards *cultural proficiency*, wherein an intrinsic understanding of cultural competency is woven into each aspect of clinical practice to provide equitable healthcare for all patients.

References

1. Hidalgo N. Multicultural teacher introspection. In T. Perry & J. W. Fraser (Eds.), Freedom's plow: teaching in the multicultural classroom. New York, NY: Routledge. 1993. p. 99–106.
2. American Psychological Association. Guidelines on multicultural education, training, research, practice, and organizational change for psychologists. Am Psychol. 2003;58(5):377.
3. National Quality Forum. A comprehensive framework and preferred practices for measuring and reporting cultural competency: a consensus report. Washington, DC: NQF; 2009. p. 116.
4. Colby SL, Ortman JM. Projections of the size and composition of the U.S. population: 2014 to 2060, Current Population Reports, P25-1143, U.S. Census Bureau, Washington, DC, 2014. https://www.census.gov/content/dam/Census/library/publications/2015/demo/p25-1143.pdf.
5. Healthy People 2020. Disparities [Web Page]. Washington, DC: ODPHP; 2010. Available from: http://www.healthypeople.gov/2020/about/disparitiesAbout.aspx.
6. US Department of Health. The Secretary's Advisory Committee on National Health Promotion and Disease Prevention Objectives for 2020. Phase I report: recommendations for the framework and format of healthy people 2020. Section IV. Advisory Committee findings and recommendations. 2008.
7. Carter-Pokras O, Baquet C. What is a "health disparity"? Public Health Rep. 2002;117(5):426–34.
8. The Patient Protection and Affordable Care Act (PPACA). USA Affordable Care Act. 2010:111–48.
9. Shaw SJ, Huebner C, Armin J, Orzech K, Vivian J. The role of culture in health literacy and chronic disease screening and management. J Immigr Minor Health. 2009;11(6):460–7.
10. Sentell T, Braun KL. Low health literacy, limited English proficiency, and health status in Asians, Latinos, and other racial/ethnic groups in California. J Health Commun. 2012;17(Suppl 3): 82–99.
11. Wilson E, Chen AHM, Grumbach K, Wang F, Fernandez A. Effects of limited English proficiency and physician language on health care comprehension. J Gen Intern Med. 2005;20(9):800–6.
12. Smith MM, Rose SH, Schroeder DR, Long TR. Diversity of United States medical students by region compared to US census data. Adv Med Educ Pract. 2015;6:367–72.

13. Van Voorhees AS, Enos CW. Diversity in dermatology residency programs. J Investig Dermatol Symp Proc. 2017;18(2):S46–S9.
14. Data USA. Physicians & Surgeons 2017. Available from: https://datausa.io/profile/soc/physicians-surgeons#demographics.
15. Pandya AG, Alexis AF, Berger TG, Wintroub BU. Increasing racial and ethnic diversity in dermatology: a call to action. J Am Acad Dermatol. 2016;74(3):584–7.
16. Kennedy BR, Mathis CC, Woods AK. African Americans and their distrust of the health care system: healthcare for diverse populations. J Cult Divers. 2007;14(2):56–60.
17. Claramita M, Dalen JV, Van Der Vleuten CPM. Doctors in a Southeast Asian country communicate sub-optimally regardless of patients' educational background. Patient Educ Couns. 2011;85(3):e169–e74.
18. Claramita M, Nugraheni MD, van Dalen J, van der Vleuten C. Doctor–patient communication in Southeast Asia: a different culture? Adv Health Sci Educ. 2013;18(1):15–31.
19. Antshel KM. Integrating culture as a means of improving treatment adherence in the Latino population. Psychol Health Med. 2002;7(4):435–49.
20. Maher P. A review of 'traditional' aboriginal health beliefs. Aust J Rural Health. 1999;7(4):229–36.
21. Flores G. Culture and the patient-physician relationship: achieving cultural competency in health care. J Pediatr. 2000;136(1):14–23.
22. World Health Organization. WHO traditional medicine strategy 2002–2005. Geneva: World Health Organization; 2002.
23. Qi Z. Who traditional medicine strategy 2014–2023. Geneva: World Health Organization; 2013.
24. Shelley BM, Sussman AL, Williams RL, Segal AR, Crabtree BF. 'They don't ask me so I don't tell them': patient-clinician communication about traditional, complementary, and alternative medicine. Ann Fam Med. 2009;7(2):139–47.
25. Parker RM, Baker DW, Williams MV, Nurss JR. The test of functional health literacy in adults: a new instrument for measuring patients' literacy skills. J Gen Intern Med. 1995;10(10):537–41.
26. National Council on Interpreting in Health Care. The terminology of healthcare interpreting: a glossary of terms. 2001:1–10. https://www.ncihc.org/assets/documents/NCIHC%20Terms%20Final080408.pdf.
27. Flores G, Abreu M, Barone CP, Bachur R, Lin H. Errors of medical interpretation and their potential clinical consequences: a

comparison of professional versus ad hoc versus no interpreters. Ann Emerg Med. 2012;60(5):545–53.

28. Kleinman A. The Illness Narratives: Suffering, healing and the human condition. Encyclopaedia of human biology. New York: Basic Books. 1988.

29. American Psychiatric Association: Diagnostic and statistical manual of mental disorders: Fifth Edition. Arlington, VA: American Psychiatric Association; 2013.

30. Baile WF, Buckman R, Lenzi R, Glober G, Beale EA, Kudelka AP. SPIKES—A six-step protocol for delivering bad news: application to the patient with cancer. Oncologist. 2000;5(4):302–11.

31. Berlin EA, Fowkes WC Jr. A teaching framework for cross-cultural health care. Application in family practice. West J Med. 1983;139(6):934–8.

Index

© The Author(s) 2021
N. A. Vashi (ed.), *Cultural Practices and Dermatoses*,
https://doi.org/10.1007/978-3-030-68992-6

Printed in the United States
by Baker & Taylor Publisher Services